D1192548

Forensic Dentistry

Publication Number 990

AMERICAN LECTURE SERIES®

A Publication in

The BANNERSTONE DIVISION *of*
AMERICAN LECTURES IN FORENSIC PATHOLOGY

Editor of the Series

RUSSELL S. FISHER, B.S., M.D.

Professor of Forensic Pathology
University of Maryland Medical School
Chief Medical Examiner
State of Maryland
Baltimore, Maryland

Forensic Dentistry

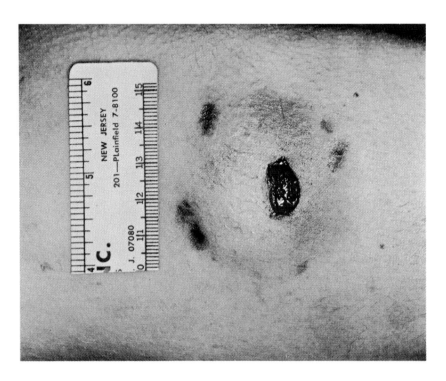

Frontispiece. Human bite mark surrounding a stab wound of the left arm of a stabbing victim. The forensic analysis of such vital evidence is further described and depicted in Chapter IX.

FORENSIC DENTISTRY

By

IRVIN M. SOPHER, D.D.S., M.D.

Deputy Chief Medical Examiner, State of Maryland

Clinical Associate Professor of Pathology
University of Maryland, School of Medicine
Baltimore, Maryland

Lecturer in Forensic Pathology
The Johns Hopkins University
School of Hygiene and Public Health
Baltimore, Maryland

Associate Professorial Lecturer
George Washington University
Department of Forensic Sciences
Washington, D. C.

Director of Research and Training
Maryland Medical-Legal Foundation, Inc.
Baltimore, Maryland

Chief Medical Examiner, State of West Virginia
Charleston, West Virginia

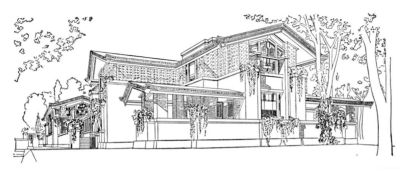

CHARLES C THOMAS · PUBLISHER
Springfield · Illinois · U.S.A.

Published and Distributed Throughout the World by
CHARLES C THOMAS • PUBLISHER
Bannerstone House
301-327 East Lawrence Avenue, Springfield, Illinois, U.S.A.

© *1976, by* CHARLES C THOMAS • PUBLISHER
ISBN 0-398-03474-5
Library of Congress Catalog Card Number: 75-14179

*With THOMAS BOOKS careful attention is given to all details of
manufacturing and design. It is the Publisher's desire to present books that are
satisfactory as to their physical qualities and artistic possibilities and
appropriate for their particular use. THOMAS BOOKS will be true to those
laws of quality that assure a good name and good will.*

Printed in the United States of America
C-1

Library of Congress Cataloging in Publication Data

Sopher, Irvin M.
    Forensic dentistry.

    (American lecture series; no. 990)
    Includes index.
    1. Dental jurisprudence. 2. Identification.
I. Title. [DNLM: 1. Forensic dentistry. W705 S712f]
RA1062.S64   614'.19   75-14179
ISBN 0-398-03474-5

to

HARLAN I. FIRMINGER, M.D.
Professor, Gentleman and Friend

PREFACE

IN RECENT YEARS, the accelerated application of scientific methodology to criminalistics and to the field of law has led to the creation and subsequent recognition of a multitude of special study disciplines which comprise the forensic sciences. Forensic dentistry, the application of dentistry to the legal structure, is relatively new in the forensic science arena. The primary focus of forensic dentistry is upon identification of unknown remains by means of the dentition. The entity of forensic dentistry occupies a primary niche within the total spectrum of methods applied to medicolegal identification. By the very nature of this organized body of expertise, it is evident that the subject matter is pertinent not only to the dental practitioner but to many other members of the scientific and legal community as well. It must be realized, therefore, that forensic dentistry is intimately related to the interests of the law enforcement officer, the forensic laboratory scientist, the physician- or lay-coroner, the anthropologist, the trial lawyer and, of course, the forensic pathologist. Furthermore, the predicted continued emphasis upon the application of science to law enforcement and, hence, to the system of justice indicates the need for a text in forensic dentistry which will be relevant to the interests of all concerned with forensic science.

This text is not only written as a compendium of the practical and academic aspects of forensic dentistry for the dentist interested in or actively engaged in the field but is also composed in the interest of the nondentist reader. Special attention has been directed toward the needs of the physician, pathologist and forensic pathologist to enable such individuals to competently engage in body identification by utilization of the dentition. Such persons can easily master the concepts involved in much the same manner as the forensic pathologist has added forensic anthropology to his armamentarium of methods for identification of the unknown body.

The initial chapter of the text introduces the reader to the forensic sciences, forensic pathology and the interrelationship of dentistry with these disciplines. Chapter II, specifically included for the nondentist reader, presents the basic anatomy and nomenclature of the teeth and the basic principles of dentistry and its materials. The third chapter concerns the panoramic format of medicolegal identification and the integrated role of dental identification. Chapter IV provides a survey of dental identification as it relates to the aircraft accident. Included is a summarization of methodology and results as reported by numerous investigators worldwide. "Basic Concepts of Dental Identification: The Antemortem Data," Chapter V, discusses the validity of the use of the teeth as a scientific method of body identification. The components of the antemortem data necessary for the dental comparison are also introduced. Chapter VI elucidates the procedural and technical aspects of the postmortem dental examination, including radiography. Included is the examination equipment, the charting procedures and the approach to the mass disaster situation. "The Postmortem Dental Data," as discussed in Chapter VII, presents the common parameters utilized in the accomplishment of the dental identification. The chapter is richly fortified with illustrative material to convey this important information. A discussion of the conclusions derived from the dental comparison ends the subject. Chapter VIII concerns general considerations as to determination of the age of unknown remains and then concentrates upon the role of the dentition as an indicator of chronologic age. The methodology for dental age estimation within the various age categories is elucidated. The final chapter, "Bite Mark Analysis," provides insight into the most controversial area of forensic dentistry. The text material introduces the general principles of bite mark comparison, discusses the interpretation of the data and presents the author's philosophy regarding the conclusions of the analysis. A consideration of the legal aspects pertinent to bite mark evidence is included. To supplement the didactic material, an actual case workup is provided.

I.M.S.

ACKNOWLEDGMENTS

I WISH TO EXPRESS my sincerest appreciation for the time and effort provided by the Medical Illustration Service of the Armed Forces Institute of Pathology. The fine work of this department enabled me to supplement the written text material with numerous illustrations. Specifically, Mr. Arthur Kluge and Mr. Oscar Rodbell were extremely helpful.

I also wish to thank the National Institute of Dental Research, National Institutes of Health, Bethesda, Maryland, for the permission and availability of several illustrations from its *Dental Science Handbook,* edited by L. W. Morrey and R. J. Nelsen.

The secretarial responsibilities of the manuscript were expertly handled by Ms. Juanita Taylor. I am also most grateful to Patrick Besant-Matthews, M.D., currently chief medical examiner of King County, Washington, for his photographic expertise and contributions. Miss Judy Conkling, a dental student, contributed numerous suggestions about the final organization of the manuscript.

In conclusion, I must not exclude the numerous law enforcement officers, physicians, dentists and students who, by their queries and continued interest in the subject, provided the impetus for the writing of the text.

CONTENTS

Forensic Dentistry

Chapter I

FORENSIC SCIENCE, FORENSIC PATHOLOGY AND THE DENTIST

THE SPECTRUM OF THE FORENSIC SCIENCES

THE RECENT, RAPID growth of the medical subspecialty of forensic pathology in this country has fostered the expansion of the allied field of forensic odontology. With an expected increase in community awareness of the services of the forensic pathologist, the demand for these medical specialists will further emphasize and catalyze the development of the field of forensic dentistry. *Forensic dentistry,* broadly defined as the application of the science of dentistry to the field of law, represents one of many fields which comprise the forensic sciences. Forensic dentistry is synonymous and interchangeable with the designation, *forensic odontology.* The spectrum of the forensic sciences, defined as any organized body of scientific knowledge or technology and its subsequent application to forensic (or legal) matters, ranges from trace evidence analysis, which deals with particulate evidence as retrieved from the scene of a crime or felony, to forensic pathology, which concerns itself with the dead body and its relationship to any subsequent legal situation. Several areas of study included in the forensic sciences are the fields of missile ballistics and tool mark comparison, analysis of questioned documents, fingerprint identification, serologic analysis of body fluids, toxicology, metallurgy and criminology. Particular areas within the forensic science spectrum which directly relate to the human subject include the fields of forensic psychiatry, forensic anthropology and dentistry, and forensic pathology. In essence, the forensic sciences are charged with the responsibility of the evaluation of evidence, based upon scientific methodology, and the relationship of such evidence to the legal frame of reference pertaining to the case at hand. It is obvious that forensic science ramifies into many independent spheres of the scientific arena, each commonly bound by their dedication to the establishment of truth.

The entity of forensic dentistry comprises four major areas of interest:

1. *Dental identification of the unknown body:* By far, this area of the field represents practically the entire body of dental case material.

2. *Bite mark comparison:* The analysis of bite mark evidence comprises a very small but very significant aspect of the field of forensic dentistry.

3. *Trauma and the oral tissues:* This area involves the interpretation of oral injury and its application to legal matters.

4. *Dental malpractice and negligence:* By definition, the opinion of the dentist who is an expert witness pertaining to such matters represents another segment of forensic dentistry.

It can be seen from the above description of the field that the dentist concerned with matters of forensic odontology is primarily relegated to an examination of human remains. The introduction of the dentist into matters concerning the dead body necessitates the interposition of a legal official who, by local law, is responsible for jurisdictional custody of the remains. Such an official is either the medical examiner or a coroner, depending upon the legal jurisdiction in question. Because the dentist concerned with the practical aspects of forensic dentistry will function under the aegis of the medical examiner or coroner system existing at the place of death, it is pertinent that he possess some knowledge regarding the various medicolegal systems established in this country which govern the disposition of the dead body. The terms, "medical examiner system" and "coroner system," are not synonymous and frequently represent quite contrasting degrees of expertise regarding the matters to be discussed. A description and comparison of these systems follows.

FORENSIC PATHOLOGY: THE MEDICAL EXAMINER SYSTEM

A forensic pathologist is a physician trained in the specialty of pathology as well as in the subspecialty of forensic pathology. Forensic pathology is a subspecialty recognized by the American Board of Pathology; eligibility to the field requires four to six years residency training beyond medical school graduation. This training includes concentrated study in the recognition of diseased tissues and organs, the effects of physical and chemical injury upon bodily structures and the relationship of disease and injury to the death of the individual.

Forensic pathology is principally concerned with the application of the science of medicine to the field of law. More specifically, the forensic pathologist deals primarily with the cause and manner of death in cases falling within his legal domain, a domain established by the local city, county or state legislation formulated to handle the medicolegal aspects of certain deaths. Such legislation, known as a medical examiner law, specifically encompasses certain types of death to best serve the interest of the citizenry as well as the legal functions of the jurisdiction. The medical examiner law establishes the legal background regarding certain specified circumstances of death and further creates a local governmental agency to expedite the medical investigation of cases that fall within the law. This agency is known as an office of the medical examiner; such an office operating within the framework of a medical examiner law comprises the medical examiner system. The forensic pathologist serves as the medical examiner.

In a general sense, a typical medical examiner law concerns *all* deaths that result from accident, suicide and homicide in addition to deaths as a result of natural causes wherein a physician was not attending the deceased.

In deaths due to natural causes (such as heart attack, stroke, pneumonia or cancer) wherein the deceased was attended by a physician, the attending physician can ascertain the manner of death as *natural,* and the case would not fall within the realm of the medical examiner law. The responsibility of certification of death in such cases is carried by the attending medical practitioner. Such deaths represent the majority of deaths occurring in the community. Deaths related to accident, homicide or suicide, or occurring under suspicious circumstances, are medical examiner cases by law and cannot be certified under any circumstances by an attending physician. Similarly, death due to apparent natural causes, but without the attendance of a physician, must be investigated and so certified by the medical examiner. In essence, such a law is promulgated to insure that all deaths within the jurisdiction are certified by a physician, the person best qualified to evaluate and thus legally certify the cause and manner of death. An undertaker cannot remove a body from a hospital or scene of death without a death certificate signed by a physician.

The following excerpt from the Medical Examiner's Act of the State of Florida[1] lists what actual cases are to be investigated in that state by the medical examiner:

> When in the State of Florida any person shall die (a) of criminal violence, (b) by accident, (c) by suicide, (d) suddenly when in apparent good health, (e) when unattended by a practicing physician or other recognized practitioner, (f) in any prison or penal institution, (g) when in police custody, (h) in any suspicious or unusual circumstance, (i) by criminal abortion, (j) by poison, (k) by disease constituting a threat to public health, (l) by disease or injury or toxic agent resulting from employment, (m) when a dead body is brought into the State of Florida without proper medical certification or (n) when a body is to be cremated, dissected or buried at sea, the medical examiner of the district in which the death occurred or the body was found shall determine the cause of death and shall make or have performed such examinations, investigations and autopsies as he shall deem necessary or as shall be requested by the

state attorney or county solicitor. The medical examiner shall have the authority in any case coming under any of the above categories to perform or have performed whatever autopsies or laboratory examinations that he deems necessary in the public interest.

The Florida Medical Examiner's Act embodies the general principles set forth in most medical examiner systems operating in this country. The medical examiner law empowers the medical examiner to carry out an investigation, including autopsies, as deemed necessary in the public interest. These laws are enacted to insure the future well-being, health and safety of the population as well as to enforce the scientific pursuit of truth and justice.

The techniques and interpretation of the medicolegal autopsy differ considerably from the routine hospital autopsy. The goal of the medicolegal autopsy is the establishment of the cause and manner of death, the interpretation of this data in relationship to the circumstances of death and the application of the results of the postmortem examination to assist in the disposition of any subsequent legal issues arising from the death.

Cause and Manner of Death

Those concerned with the legal aspects of death must be familiar with the concept of cause and manner of death. The terms, *cause of death* and *manner of death,* are especially confusing to many persons and are often incorrectly regarded as synonymous. The cause of death pertains to the pathologic entity directly responsible for death (e.g. heart disease, cancer of the lung, multiple injuries, gunshot wound of the heart, conflagration). The term represents the disease or injury considered responsible for death. The manner of death is a medicolegal classification based upon the postmortem findings and the circumstances surrounding the death. It represents the manner in which the cause of death transpired. The classification of manner of death includes five categories:

1. Natural—death occurring from natural disease processes, such as heart disease, cancer, pneumonia, etc.

2. Accident—death as a result of household, vehicular, occupational or other accidental injuries.

3. Suicide—the voluntary or intentional taking of one's own life.

4. Homicide—the death of one individual due to the purposeful or negligent actions of another person.

5. Undetermined—a category comprising a small percentage of cases wherein the manner of death cannot be ascertained despite thorough, naked-eye, microscopic and toxicologic analyses of the tissues as well as a complete investigation of the circumstances surrounding death. In other

instances, the cause of death may be quite evident (e.g. gunshot wound in the head); however, the manner of death may be undetermined.

The interrelationship of the terms *cause of death* and *manner of death* are illustrated in the following examples:

1. A 48-year-old man is found dead in bed with a gunshot wound in the head. Upon completion of the postmortem examination, the pathologist notes the cause of death to be a *close range* gunshot wound in the head. The manner of death can only be determined by a thorough investigation of the scene of death as well as the circumstances surrounding the death. Is there evidence to suggest that the deceased took his own life (suicide)? Was the deceased shot by another person (homicide)? Does evidence support any possibility that the weapon discharged accidentally (accident)?

2. A body is discovered on the sidewalk adjacent to a six-story building. The cause of death is attributed to multiple injuries including a broken neck. The manner of death is dependent upon scene evidence indicating whether the deceased jumped (suicide), was intentionally pushed (homicide) or fell (accident) out of the window.

3. A 63-year-old man was involved in a minor vehicular traffic accident wherein he sustained no bodily injury. The subject became quite irate and excited over the accident and one hour later complained of severe chest pain and fatally collapsed. Postmortem examination disclosed marked coronary arteriosclerosis (hardening of the arteries of the heart) as the cause of death. Although this cause of death represents a natural disease process, the accessory facts that (a) a period of sudden undue stress and excitement are known to precipitate a fatal heart attack and (b) the fatal attack chronologically ensued shortly after the traffic accident, establish the manner of death as *accident*.

4. The autopsy examination of a woman who fatally collapsed during a purse-snatching disclosed marked coronary arteriosclerosis as the cause of death. Despite the extent of heart disease, the subject died as a direct result of the circumstances surrounding the robbery. The occurrence of death due to a natural disease process, but precipitated by a felony, results in the designation of the manner of death as *homicide*.

5. An elderly farmer falls to the floor while carrying a kerosene lantern into the barn. The subsequent conflagration engulfs the victim. Autopsy examination discloses a recent brain hemorrhage as a result of high blood pressure, as well as extensive body burns. The absence of carbon monoxide (carboxyhemoglobin) in the blood or soot in the airway upon postmortem examination indicates that the victim had died prior to the onset of the fire. The medical facts in the case indicate that the deceased died of a natural disease process prior to the subsequent conflagration. Despite the initial suggestion that death was accidental, the autopsy disclosed that the cause of death was a stroke and the manner of death is designated as *natural*.

6. A 32-year-old male pedestrian received lower extremity fractures as a result of being struck by an automobile. Despite an apparently uncomplicated recuperative period, the patient suddenly expired during the fifth week of his hospitalization. The postmortem examination disclosed that the cause of death was pulmonary embolism, a condition whereby a fatal blood clot forms in the leg or pelvic veins and travels to the lung. This embolic phenomenon, a known

complication of such an injury, indicates that death was related to the injury which occurred five weeks earlier, and the manner of death is designated as *accident*.

Each of the above examples represent typical case material found within any medical examiner's office. The responsibility of the forensic pathologist is to certify the cause and manner of death based upon the data revealed by both the postmortem examination and the circumstances surrounding the death. Further, it is the duty of the forensic pathologist to present the scientific evidence regarding his findings in a court of law, if necessary.

The derivation of the manner of death is important in that it serves as a guideline for other parties interested in any particular death. Police personnel are initially concerned about the manner of death since this designation determines the subsequent course of their investigation. The state's attorney office is concerned with homicidal and accidental or suicidal deaths. Numerous industrial and governmental organizations may be interested in accidental deaths of various types in an effort to improve the man-environment relationship. Deaths classified as *natural* represent sources of data for local health agencies in their assessment of various epidemiologic aspects of disease. Needless to say, cases involving any manner of death and all causes of death may involve the necessity of dental expertise. The spectrum of the dentist may range from dental identification (all manners of death) to bite mark analysis (homicide cases) and would include the interpretation of oral injuries as well as the dental aspects of a fatality occurring during or as a result of dental treatment. In such instances the dentist is charged with the responsibility of investigation as well as the incorporation of his data as a legal document within the official autopsy protocol. In addition, the dentist may be expected to testify in court regarding his findings.

The importance of a medical examiner system is appreciated when one realizes that in jurisdictions governed by a medical examiner law, approximately 25 percent of all deaths occurring within the jurisdiction fall within the medical examiner statute. For the year 1972, for example, the Office of the Medical Examiner, State of Maryland, was responsible for certification of 7,372 of the 32,826 total deaths occurring within that state. Table I discloses the percentage distribution of the manners of death at that office for the same year. These figures are representative of other medical examiner systems throughout the country.

In the mind of the layman, the forensic pathologist or medical examiner is primarily associated with homicide, and the connotation of *city morgue* with bizarre murder cases has been historically perpetuated

TABLE I

MANNER OF DEATH, OFFICE OF THE CHIEF MEDICAL EXAMINER,
STATE OF MARYLAND, FOR THE YEAR 1972*

	No. of Cases	Percent of Total Cases
Natural	4,497	60.9
Accident	1,768	23.9
Homicide	521	7.1
Suicide	473	6.4
Undetermined	113	1.5
Total	7,372	99.8

* From the *Thirty-Fourth Annual Report,* Office of the Chief Medical Examiner, State of Maryland.

through the years. In truth, however, such cases represent only about 6 percent of the total caseload of a medical examiner facility. While it is true that much notoriety is afforded the medical examiner due to the mass communication media which report such crimes, these cases represent but a small fragment of the total contribution by a medical examiner system to the community when one considers the total functions of such an agency.

The assignment of the correct manner of death in any case is of paramount importance to interested parties. Surviving family members may benefit from accidental deaths. Workmen's compensation benefits may be applicable to other instances of natural or accidental deaths under certain circumstances. The analysis of injury patterns and cause of death in industrial, vehicular and aircraft accidents, when coupled with the scene investigation, can lead to improvement in safety and design regarding the man-machine relationship. Similar evaluation and investigation of fatal home accidents also contribute to improving man's relationship with his environment. Common examples of the latter are deaths due to electrocution, fire and carbon monoxide poisoning. It must be emphasized that, in addition to the legal implications inherent in an accident case, the postmortem investigation of the accidental death is designed to assist in the prevention of future similar accidents. Within the sphere of natural deaths, which constitute approximately 60 to 70 percent of the medical examiner office's caseload, not only is the cause of death certified, but disease patterns may be recognized which represent important contributions to the epidemiologic aspects of disease. Occupational and pollution-related diseases as well as unsuspected environmental poisons may so be identified and corrected. Previously undetected genetic and infectious diseases may also be documented, which can lead to the institution of preventive health measures for surviving family members.

The medical examiner system provides an important focus for medical research in the specialized areas of pathology, trauma and toxicology. It also serves as a nidus for research activity in the various fields of forensic science, criminology and public health.

The identification of unknown human remains represents another vital area within the realm of forensic pathology, a segment of which is covered in the greater part of this book.

The training and experience of the forensic pathologist attune him with and direct him toward community medical and medicolegal problems as mentioned above. It is quite obvious that jurisdictions which operate without such a system are deprived of vital information pertinent to the surviving family, the community, the field of medicine, interested law enforcement agencies and the judiciary system.

A common misconception regarding medical examiner systems is that these organizations represent an extension of the law enforcement agencies. Such an impression is a false one. A medical examiner system represents and protects the public. The findings of the forensic pathologist represent the ultimate effort in the search for truth regarding cause and manner of death and, further, concerning the exploration of the relationship between the death and the community. An office of the medical examiner is a neutral scientific agency established by law to gather and interpret the medical facts pertinent to the death in question. The fact of death is a very legal issue in our modern society. The dead should be afforded the same degree of medical attention as the living.

MEDICAL EXAMINER SYSTEMS VS. CORONER SYSTEMS IN THE UNITED STATES

Despite the benefits that accrue to the population from the establishment of a medical examiner system, it has been estimated that, at most, only one third to one half of this nation's citizenry are protected by medical examiner laws.[2] In contrast, many states and/or large segments thereof still possess outmoded coroner systems. Many of these coroner jurisdictions, whether at state, county or city level, are staffed by a nonphysician coroner who is primarily responsible for the ultimate decision regarding cause and manner of death. In many instances, the coroner is an elected official whose primary occupation may be that of an undertaker, pharmacist, lawyer, sheriff or carpenter. It is rather obvious that such individuals cannot provide the expertise required for the settlement of the often complex medical and legal issues that arise from deaths occurring under their jurisdiction. Other jurisdictions possess a coroner system controlled by a physician. The latter format represents a step in the right direction; however, the nonforensic pathologist-physician is also neither trained nor qualified in the matters of forensic pathology. The optimal situation is the

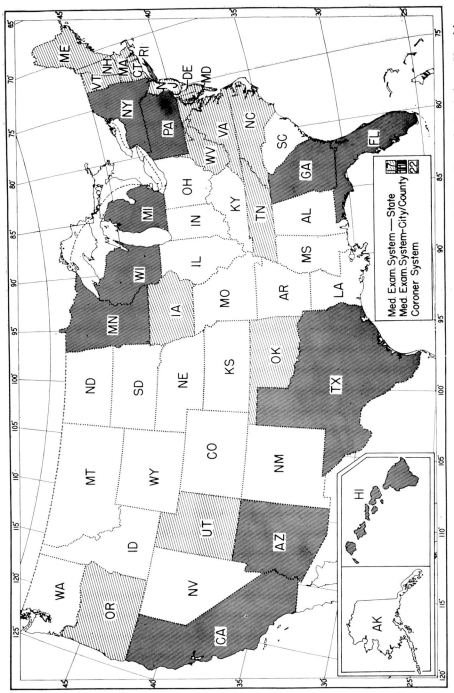

Figure 1. Distribution of the various medicolegal systems in the United States as of 1971. Data derived from Kornblum, R. N. and Fisher, R. S.[3] AFIP Neg. No. 72-17846.

Legend:
Med. Exam. System—State
Med. Exam. System-City/County
Coroner System

creation of a medical examiner system operating under a medical examiner law and staffed by one or more forensic pathologists.

The nationwide distribution of medical examiner vs. coroner systems is depicted in Figure 1.[3] A tabulation of states discloses that only seventeen states possess a legislated operational medical examiner system embodying a uniform statewide law which applies to the entire population of that particular state. Twelve states operate under medical examiner legislation which pertains only to varying segments of the state population. These states possess operating medical examiner systems at substate levels; that is, individual counties or cities may have established medical examiner structures; however, the neighboring counties are under coroner systems. A total of twenty-one states are governed by coroner laws only, without benefit of any medical examiner legislation. Needless to say, the majority of such coroner agencies have proven totally inadequate for the assigned mission of protecting the public welfare and safety.

The article by Luke, Sturner and Petty[2] reveals some quite poignant statistics emphasizing the misclassification of cause and manner of death in areas under coroner jurisdiction. Only recently have the citizenry, law enforcement officials, the judiciary and legislators become aware of the importance of the proper medicolegal investigation of community deaths. Such enlightenment has been fostered by several violent deaths of national importance (the Kennedy brothers and Martin Luther King assassinations, the Attica Prison riot deaths and the Los Angeles Symbionese Liberation Army house fire). This delayed, but rapidly developing appreciation of the importance of the field of forensic pathology has resulted in a recent expansion in the number of statewide or local medical examiner systems as well as revision of some existing coroner offices.

The above discussion of the varied legislation regarding jurisdiction of the dead body sets the stage upon which the dentist, interested in forensic dentistry, may find himself occupying a leading role.

ENTRY OF THE DENTIST INTO THE FORENSIC SCIENCES

By virtue of the existing legislation governing the control and disposition of the dead body, the forensic dentist must function under the aegis of the established medical examiner or coroner serving his geographic area of interest. The dentist must remember that the field of forensic dentistry represents an unknown commodity in most areas of the country. This statement especially applies to coroner jurisdictions. The established medical examiner systems have generally evolved within and surrounding the larger metropolitan centers of our country. Such metropolitan medical examiner offices currently represent the locations wherein the majority of the nation's forensic pathologists are concentrated. In contrast to the coroner the forensic pathologist deals with medicolegal situations as his primary occupation, an occupation which represents the culmination of several years of training focused upon the complex medicolegal problems encountered in society every day. As a result of his specialized training and experience, the forensic pathologist is quite cognizant of the interaction between his field of endeavor and the other areas included in the totality of forensic science. The forensic pathologist or medical examiner is well aware of the value and application of forensic dentistry. One appreciates this fact when one considers that most of the medical examiner systems in this country have one or more forensic dentists as consultant members of their staff.

In contradistinction, the coroner system possesses less expertise relevant to the problems under consideration. This not only applies to the more routine encounters with such matters as cause and manner of death but is especially applicable to the more erudite ramifications of the forensic sciences including forensic dentistry. The point to be emphasized is that there is a great need across the country for dental expertise relevant to forensic dentistry. This need is particularly acute in the setting of the coroner system and even more so in the more rural communities of such jurisdictions. Despite the progressive increase in dissemination of knowledge regarding the forensic sciences to law enforcement personnel, in a parallel sense the smaller community police departments also disclose a lack of realization regarding the potential contributions of forensic dentistry. The fact of the matter is that where unfamiliarity with the spectrum of forensic science exists, an appreciation of what is potentially available in the field is also lacking.

The dentist should realize that due to the above-discussed situation, one can hardly expect the local sheriff or coroner to parade to his doorstep bearing fragments of a maxilla or mandible as components of an unidentified body. It is the responsibility of the dentist to make his presence and interest known to local officials so that his expertise can be utilized when necessary. The dentist must assume the initiative and offer his services. In the process his missionary role will hopefully foster the education of law enforcement and coroner officials pertaining to the realm of dental identification. In this manner the local general practitioner of dentistry can offer his knowledge in satisfying a vital legal and humane function applicable to the welfare of his community.

The above discussion of the potential and existing need for application of dental knowledge to the forensic sciences is not meant to imply that even the well established medical examiner facilities are adequately staffed with dental consultants. The availability of an interested forensic dentist is a valuable asset to any such facility. Again, the need for such assistance in any particular location can only be assayed by personal inquiry. One finds that the ready availability of an interested dentist greatly enhances the utilization of his services by the consulting agency. Close rapport between the two parties results in an educational experience for the medical staff and leads to increased utilization of the consultant dentist. The end result is maximum application of forensic science to the problem at hand, whether it be identification or analysis of bite mark evidence. Every medical examiner or coroner system should strive to establish and maintain such a standard.

The actual number of cases requiring dental consultation in the active practice of forensic pathology is not great. The significance of the contribution of forensic dentistry does not rest in numbers but in the extreme importance of the expertise in those cases to which it applies. This is to say that very frequently the only means of specific identification rests within the dentition. Similarly, bite mark evidence is certainly more rarely encountered; however, the proper analysis of the case may be of paramount importance in the instrumentation of justice. The Medical Examiner's Office of the State of Maryland examines approximately 3,800 to 4,000 bodies per year as dictated by the state's medical examiner law. Of this total caseload, about seventy-five cases per year require the application of dental expertise. Almost all of these instances involve the dental identification of unknown remains. Having been personally associated with the Maryland system intermittently for several years, the author can state that this represents the maximum figure for this particular facility. A similar ratio of dental consultations per caseload should exist in other medical examiner systems throughout the country, provided a dentist is consulted in every case where his knowledge should be utilized. It must be remembered that, all too often, the governing official responsible for certifying the identification may accept less reliable means of identification without calling upon the dental profession. This statement especially applies to coroner establishments. The truth of the matter is that it is the responsibility of the system, be it a coroner or medical examiner organization, to provide a modern application of technology to the problem at hand. Intelligent insight regarding the potential contribution of forensic dentistry to the matters under discussion is representative of modern technology and science. The absence of such an appreciation borders upon the archaic.

The law enforcement agencies, coroners and medical examiners are not solely to blame for the dearth of forensic dental consultants. Some of the blame rests on the members of the dental profession themselves. This country lags far behind Scandinavia, Great Britain and Japan in the recognition of and contribution to the field of forensic dentistry. Not until 1969 was the American Society of Forensic Odontology established, and in 1970 an Odontology Section was formed within the American Academy of Forensic Sciences. Even in 1974 only a very small number of our nation's dental schools provided any introduction to the field in their curricula. This is ironic since the dental schools, the core of dental education and research, should represent the keystone in the implementation of dental knowledge to forensic science.

While any dentist possesses the knowledge necessary to effect a dental identification, the dental school staff member is particularly suited regarding an interest in forensic dentistry since he is more likely to have the time required for an immediate response to consultation as well as for a possible subsequent appearance in the courtroom. The busy private practitioner is less likely to be able to alter an already demanding schedule to fit these requirements. In addition, the academician is in close contact with readily available specialist consultation and library material, if necessary.

The dentist should not feel hesitant about his professional competence regarding the forensic aspects of dentistry. Any dentist is qualified to concern himself with forensic dentistry because the problems encountered merely represent an extension of basic knowledge which he utilizes in his everyday practice. There are no organized residency programs in the field of forensic odontology, nor are they necessary. An excellent annual four-day course concerning the field is offered by the Armed Forces Institute of Pathology, Washington, D.C. It is the only program of such high caliber, to the author's knowledge, in the country.

It is hoped that the private dental practitioner, the dental school staff member or the local dental society as a unit will accept the challenge inherent to the field of forensic dentistry and step forward to offer knowledge for the benefit of the community.

The Dentist/Medical Examiner/Coroner Relationship

Most dental consultants to coroner or medical examiner facilities operate on a fee-for-service basis. Some consultant dentists receive no fee for their contribution and devote their efforts in exchange for interest and self-gratification. The reader should keep in mind that smaller jurisdictions do not require frequent dental consultation. The author does not foresee the need for full-time specialists concerned only with matters of forensic dentistry. Existing medical examiner or coroner systems are budgeted much like other government agencies; and the infrequent, although vital, need for legal dental expertise does not justify a salary commensurate with the expectations of the dentist. The dental manpower is available and rests within the nidus of community dentists and the teaching institutions. The problem is in urging the dentist to contribute and to acquaint the responsible officials with the need and benefits of his services.

Any association between the forensic dental consultant and the state, county or city coroner, or medical examiner agency is not without possible legal complications in itself. Such complications include the following:

1. The dentist will be in occasional contact with bodies possessing potentially contagious diseases (such as tuberculosis, meningitis, hepatitis, staphylococcal infections), and the possibility of an examiner acquiring an infection is not to be totally dismissed. In addition, the dentist may be required to frequent a scene of death which may present hazardous conditions capable of causing personal injury. The personal legal aspects of such rare but possible sequelae of a dental consultant's position should be elucidated at the time any such appointment is consummated.

2. The dentist need not be concerned with a legal charge of assault upon a dead body (as brought by next of kin) since his work would be under the auspices of the responsible medical examiner/coroner agency. Such agencies, by law, have complete jurisdiction over the remains regardless of family wishes.

3. It is advisable in bite mark cases, wherein dental impressions are effected upon a living suspect, that either a court order be issued or a voluntary consent form by the suspect be obtained to eliminate the possibility of an assault charge being levied against the dentist (see Chap. IX).

4. The potential grounds for a dental malpractice suit as a result of dental misidentification would be a unique occurrence in this country. Provided due care were exercised by the dentist in formulating his opinion, the author does not see where such a suit could evolve through the courts as a nondefensible position.

5. On occasion, a forensic dentist may be called upon for consultation in a case within a neighboring state in which the dentist does not possess a license to practice. The requirement of licensure does not apply to such a consultant relationship since the act does not represent the practice of dentistry even if a fee is received for services.

Chapter II

BASIC DENTAL ANATOMY: GENERAL PRINCIPLES OF DENTISTRY AND DENTAL MATERIALS

DENTAL ANATOMY

Development of the Dentition

Embryologic Growth

Tooth development begins during the sixth week of embryonic life (11mm embryo) with the formation of the primordial tooth buds. These primordial buds originate as a result of differential growth of the oral epithelium at loci of the dental anlage. The tooth germ develops from ectoderm and mesoderm. The former eventually gives rise to enamel; the latter differentiates into the dental pulp and dentin, the cementum and the periodontal ligament. The tooth bud originates as a proliferative invagination of the ectodermal oral epithelium with subsequent histodifferentiation of the adjacent mesodermal mesenchyme. The oral epithelium differentiates into enamel-producing ameloblasts, and the dentin-producing odontoblasts arise from the mesoderm. The dental pulp consists of mesodermal loose connective tissue, blood vessels and nerves which develop centrally within the outer tooth shell composed of dentin and enamel. The invaginating tooth buds eventually separate from the overlying oral epithelium and continue development within the gradually encompassing, concomitantly forming bone tissue representative of the mandible and maxilla. The incisor, canine and premolar permanent tooth buds, responsible for the development of these members of the secondary dentition (permanent teeth), sequester from the deciduous or primary buds during the fourth month of uterine life. At about the seventeenth week *in utero*, the tooth buds of the twelve permanent molars (six for each jaw or dental arch) develop as invaginations of the oral epithelium totally independent of the deciduous tooth buds. The anlage for the permanent teeth remain dormant until initiation of the growth process responsible for their development.

17

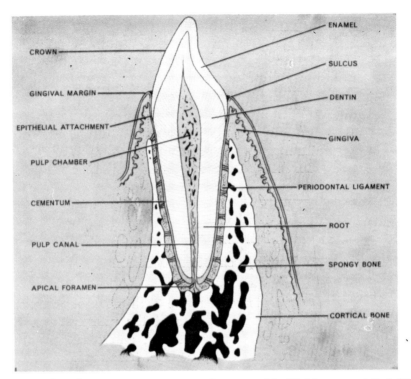

Figure 2. The dental tissues in cross-section. Courtesy of L. W. Morrey and R. J. Nelsen, *Dental Science Handbook* (U.S. Government Printing Office, 1970).

The completed definitive tooth is anatomically divided into two regions: a root (or roots) which serves as a means of stabilizing the tooth within the jaw; and a crown, that part of an erupted tooth which is visible within the mouth. The crown consists of thick walls composed of two independent homogeneous layers, an outer layer of enamel and an inner layer of dentin. The inner dentin layer encloses a third component of the crown, the central pulp chamber which contains pulpal tissue (Fig. 2).

Composition of the Tooth

Dental enamel, which comprises the external portion of the crown of the tooth, is the hardest tissue in the human body. Mature enamel is comprised of inorganic mineral salt (96%), predominantly calcium and phosphorous, with a small amount of organic substances and water (4%). The specific function of enamel is to form a resistant outer structure for the tooth crown, thereby enabling the tooth to withstand the force and abrasive action of mastication.

The bulk of the tooth structure is composed of dentin, a substance slightly harder than bone but considerably softer than enamel. The enamel of the tooth completely overlays the softer dentin within the crown portion of the tooth; and cementum, to be discussed below, covers the dentin throughout the root portion of the tooth. Dentin consists of 70 percent inorganic material, predominantly calcium and phosphorus, and 30 percent organic substances and water. The lower mineral content of dentin imparts a greater degree of radiolucency as compared to enamel on the dental X ray. Once the outer barrier of enamel is destroyed, the relatively high organic composition of dentin allows rapid penetration and spread of dental decay (caries) (see Fig. 3).

The dental pulp is a loose connective tissue which occupies the central pulp chamber and the pulp canal within the root structure of the tooth. The pulp contains vascular and neural elements which serve a nutritive and neural sensory function for the adjacent dentin layer. The nerve and blood supply of the pulp enter the tooth through the small apical foramen (or foramina in multirooted teeth) located at the root tip(s) or apex of the tooth.

Cementum is a calcified tissue of mesodermal origin which covers the root structure and furnishes a means of attachment for connective tissue fibers which secure the root of the tooth to the surrounding bony socket known as the alveolus. Cementum is softer than dentin and is composed of approximately 50 percent inorganic calcium and phosphorus and 50 percent organic material.

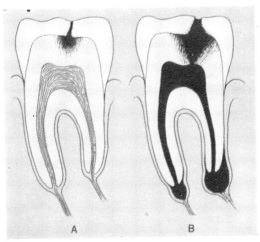

Figure 3. The progress of dental decay. A. The decay is limited to enamel and dentin, and restoration of the tooth is the indicated treatment. B. A more extensive stage of caries. The pulp has been involved, and apical abscesses are noted. The indicated treatment is root canal therapy or extraction of the tooth. Courtesy of Morrey and Nelsen, *Dental Science Handbook.*

Calcification of the Dentition

Calcification or mineralization of the developing tooth begins at the cuspal or incisal tips and proceeds rootward (towards the apex or apical foramen of the root) as the root structure develops. Due to the growth and eruption sequence of teeth, the crown is fully calcified as it emerges (erupts) through the epithelium of the gum tissues; at this time calcification of the root structures is just beginning. This concept is important when one considers age determination based upon the eruption and calcification sequence as interpreted from oral roentgenograms. Indeed, cuspal or incisal tip calcification may begin three to five years prior to eruption of the tooth into the oral cavity. For example, it is not uncommon at birth to see calcification of the cuspal regions of the first permanent molar, a tooth not scheduled to erupt until the age of six years. Complete apical root calcification of this tooth may not be noted until age ten. The rather precise progressive cusp-to-apex calcification pattern of teeth constitutes the reason why tooth development surpasses other anthropologic methods for the determination of chronologic age in persons less than fourteen years of age (see Chap. VIII).

The Primary and Secondary Dentitions

Two sets of teeth comprise the human dentition. These consist of a deciduous (primary or baby) dentition and the permanent or secondary (adult) dentition. The deciduous dentition, totaling twenty teeth, begins eruption between six to nine months of age with deciduous eruption usually complete by two to two and one-half years of age. Complete root maturation for the deciduous dentition is usually seen by three years of age. The deciduous dentition consists of five teeth per quadrant consisting of a central and a lateral incisor, the canine and a first and a second deciduous molar. The primary dentition does not contain premolars as noted in the permanent dentition (Fig. 4).

At birth and during the first several years following birth, the permanent teeth begin to calcify within the jaw bone. The permanent dentition, consisting of thirty-two teeth, enters the eruption phase at about six years of age with the emergence of the first four permanent molars (six-year molars). The specific chronologic details and further discussion of tooth eruption are considered in Chapter VIII. The complete permanent dentition contains eight teeth per quadrant: a central and a lateral incisor; a canine (cuspid); the first and second premolars (bicuspids); and first, second and third molars (Fig. 5). The permanent incisors, canines and premolars erupt into the locations previously occupied by the deciduous in-

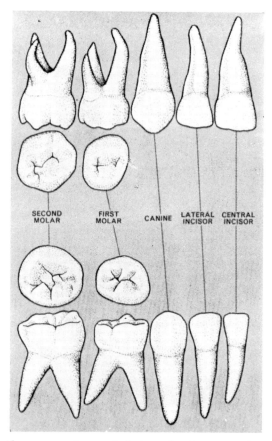

Figure 4. The deciduous or primary (baby) teeth. Courtesy of Morrey and Nelsen, *Dental Science Handbook.*

cisors, canines and molars, respectively. The permanent molars erupt at locations distal or posterior to the second deciduous molars and do not re- place deciduous teeth. In addition, the incisors and canines are known as anterior teeth; the premolars and molars are known as posterior teeth.

The reader should remember that tooth formation is a dynamic process which originates during embryonic life with differential growth and se- quential calcification of both the primary and permanent dentitions occur- ring within the respective jaws. The pressure resulting from growth and enlargement of the underlying permanent tooth crowns induces resorption of the root structure of the deciduous teeth resulting in the sequential loss of the primary dentition. If the permanent tooth bud fails to develop, the overlying deciduous tooth may be retained for life. The continuing root development of the emerging permanent tooth then gradually positions the permanent tooth in its intraoral location. Between the ages of six and

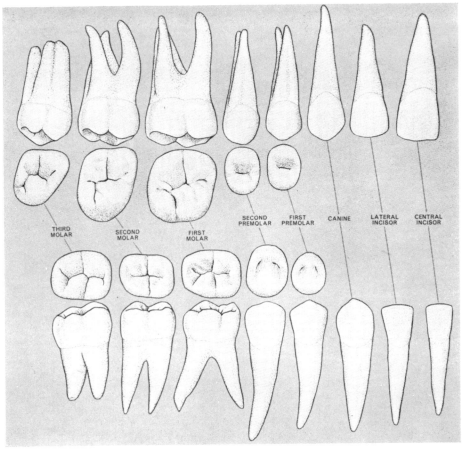

Figure 5. The adult or permanent dentition. Courtesy of Morrey and Nelsen, *Dental Science Handbook.*

fourteen years, the total complement of twenty deciduous teeth (incisors, canines and molars) are replaced by twenty permanent teeth (incisors, canines and premolars). The first and second permanent molars erupt at about six and twelve years of age, respectively. The third permanent molar (wisdom tooth) erupts at about seventeen to twenty-two years of age.

Dental Numbering Systems

In practice, the dentist utilizes a numbering system for tooth designation rather than the more cumbersome anatomic designation, such as *maxillary right second premolar*. Dentists throughout the world utilize many different numbering systems and symbols for the dentition, and the person concerned with a dental identification case need not be confused by the variety of systems employed. When discussing a case with an attending

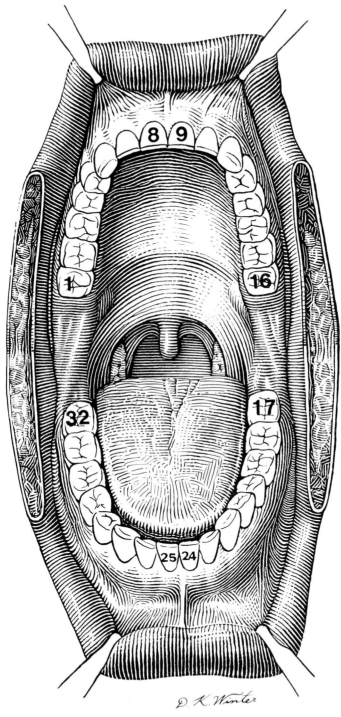

Figure 6. The Universal System of tooth designation applied to the permanent dentition. AFIP No. 65-5392-1.

TABLE II

THE UNIVERSAL SYSTEM FOR TOOTH DESIGNATION

| *Right* | | | *Left* | |
Lower	*Upper*		*Upper*	*Lower*
No. 32	No. 1	Third molars	No. 16	No. 17
No. 31	No. 2	Second molars	No. 15	No. 18
No. 30	No. 3	First molars	No. 14	No. 19
No. 29	No. 4	Second premolars	No. 13	No. 20
No. 28	No. 5	First premolars	No. 12	No. 21
No. 27	No. 6	Canines	No. 11	No. 22
No. 26	No. 7	Lateral incisors	No. 10	No. 23
No. 25	No. 8	Central incisors	No. 9	No. 24

dentist, one should be sure to establish his numbering system. Most patient dental charts, if submitted for comparison, will contain a diagram of the dentition and the corresponding tooth numbers. A commonly used numbering system in the United States is the Universal System, in which the upper right third molar is designated as number 1, the upper left third molar as number 16, the lower left third molar as number 17 and the lower right third molar as number 32. This numbering system is depicted in Figure 6 and further elucidated in Table II. If a communication problem develops, one can always give the full name of the tooth, e.g. upper right second premolar (rather than tooth number 4). Designation of the primary dentition also varies among dentists. Commonly, alphabetical letters or the permanent tooth location or number in conjunction with a D (for deciduous) is utilized for this purpose.

Tooth Surface Nomenclature

The crown of the tooth presents five surfaces upon intraoral visual examination, much like a cube or upright rectangle resting upon a flat surface. Knowledge of the particular tooth surfaces is an important aspect of dental identification because dental restorations (fillings, etc.) and caries are designated according to the surface or surfaces involved. The tooth surfaces are named in the following manner (Fig. 7):

1. The *occlusal* (O) surface is that surface of the posterior teeth which contacts the opposite tooth when the jaws are closed. It can be regarded as the masticating or chewing surface of the tooth. On anterior teeth, this surface is quite reduced in size and is referred to as the *incisal* (I) surface or edge.

2 and 3. The two tooth surfaces in direct contact with the adjacent teeth are known as the interproximal surfaces and are designated as the *mesial* (M) and *distal* (D) surfaces. These surfaces are named according to their

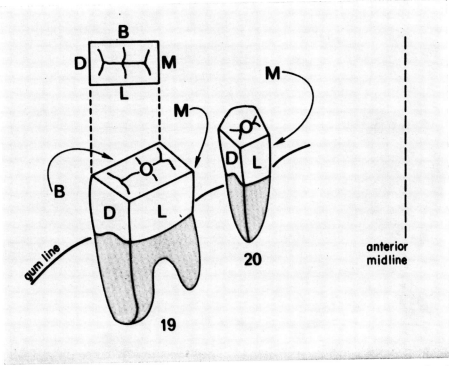

Figure 7. The anatomic designation of tooth surfaces. The view is from inside the mouth looking out, and the diagram indicates the lower left first molar (19) and second premolar (20). An artefactitious space is introduced between the two teeth for purposes of clarity. See text for description. O: occlusal; M: mesial; D: distal; B: buccal; L: lingual.

relationship with the anterior midline of the jaw. The mesial surface is that surface of the tooth directed toward or nearest to the midline of the dental arch. The distal surface faces away from the arch midline.

4 and 5. The two remaining surfaces are those which face the cheek (for posterior teeth) or lips (for anterior teeth) and the tongue. The surface of posterior teeth directed toward the cheek is the *buccal* (B) surface; this corresponds to the *labial* (LA) surface of anterior teeth. The inward surface of all teeth is the *lingual* (L) surface.

The letters M, O, D, B and L refer to mesial, occlusal, distal, buccal and lingual respectively and are utilized in dental records or in conversation with a dentist. Similarly, the letters I and LA refer to the incisal and labial surfaces of the anterior teeth. The filling material or caries activity noted on any given tooth are described according to the altered tooth surfaces. For example, a single-surface occlusal amalgam (silver) restoration on a molar would be designated as *an occlusal (O) amalgam on tooth number*. . . . A more complex continuous restoration involving two surfaces would represent a mesio-occlusal (MO), disto-occlusal (DO), occluso-buccal (OB), occluso-lingual (OL) or disto-incisal (DI), etc. depending on the involved surfaces. One can even have more extensive restorations involving three or even all five crown surfaces. Such an example would be *an MOD amalgam on tooth number* . . . , which designates a continuous silver restoration involving the mesio-occluso-distal surfaces of the particular tooth. Similarly, an MODBL restoration would represent a mesio-occluso-distal restoration with continuous buccal and lingual extensions. Two separate, independent restorations on a single tooth, such as an MO amalgam and a noncontinuous, separate buccal surface amalgam would be called *an MO amalgam and a B amalgam*. Caries designation follows the same pattern, e.g. *distal caries on number*. . . . In summary, the restorations in the mouth are designated by tooth number, surface(s) involved and type of filling or restorative material.

BASIC DENTAL PRINCIPLES, PROCEDURES AND MATERIALS
Dental Decay and Its Treatment

Dental caries (decay, cavity) represents progressive destruction of tooth structure due to bacterial acid formation. Certain types of bacteria possess the ability to convert simple sugars and other carbohydrates into acids capable of inducing demineralization of the inorganic constituents and destruction of the organic components of tooth structure. The areas of the tooth most susceptible to carious activity are the difficult-to-clean interproximal surfaces and the small pits and fissures of the occlusal surfaces. The process is progressive and irreversible with rapid destruction of the softer dentin once the enamel layer is perforated. The end results of untreated caries are involvement and death of the pulpal tissue with possible subsequent periapical (surrounding the root apex) abscess formation. Such an abscess may perforate the alveolar process of the respective jaw bone and drain into the oral cavity or drain externally via sinus tract to the face. Depending upon its duration, the periapical inflammatory process may present a small radiolucent area on the oral X ray (see Fig. 3).

Although usually symptomatic, pulpal involvement and abscess formation may develop quite insidiously and not create a degree of discomfort sufficient to cause the subject to seek dental attention. As with any bacterial infection, the course of events following pulpal involvement is dependent upon bacteria-host interaction. Death of the pulpal tissue must be treated by root canal therapy or extraction of the tooth. Root canal treatment (the specialty of endodontia) involves the removal of the necrotic pulpal

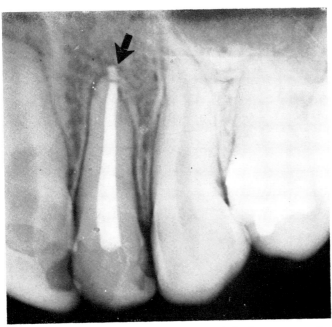

Figure 8. Oral X ray of the right upper lateral incisor (7) showing completed root canal therapy. Note the radiopaque filling material of the central pulp chamber and canal. Also note the extrusion of filling material (arrow) from the apical foramen. Such a finding represents a very specific point for comparison in dental identification. AFIP No. 73-3950-1.

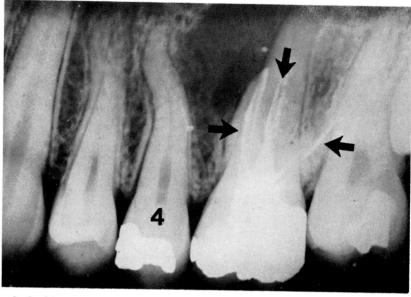

Figure 9. Oral X ray of the right upper first molar (3) depicting root canal therapy of all three roots (arrows). Notice the unusual curvature of the second premolar (4). These two findings illustrate the value of the X ray in elucidating points of comparison not visible on naked-eye examination of the mouth. AFIP No. 73-3950-2.

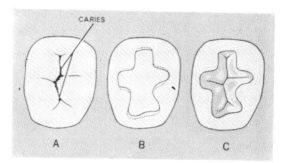

Figure 10. Cavity preparation for a molar occlusal surface amalgam restoration. Courtesy of Morrey and Nelsen, *Dental Science Handbook*.

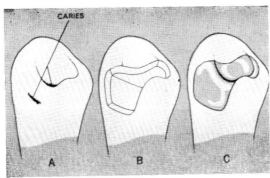

Figure 11. Cavity preparation for a premolar mesio-occlusal (MO) two-surface continuous restoration. Courtesy of Morrey and Nelsen, *Dental Science Handbook*.

material, chemical sterilization of the pulp chamber and root or pulp canal(s), and insertion of silver or nonmetallic cones into the root canals. Endodontic treatment of a tooth can only be documented by the oral X ray which nicely depicts the opaque cones and cements used in the filling of the root canal (Figs. 8 and 9). The external crown aspect of the tooth possessing root canal treatment is usually restored by one of the restorations described below, preferably a complete crown. Root canal therapy is expensive, certainly more costly than extraction of the tooth, and therefore, is not a common procedure. Because of this fact, it bears a degree of specificity regarding dental identification. The procedure may be performed on any tooth.

One of the purposes of periodic dental examination is to detect and arrest dental caries in its earliest stages. The detection of caries is followed by the removal of the carious focus and restoration of the structure and, hence, the function of the tooth. Dental instrumentation eliminates the caries-destroyed tooth structure so as to retain the restorative material to be used in tooth reconstruction. The alteration of tooth structure performed by the dentist to allow retention of the restorative material in adherence to the laws of stress and strain is known as a cavity *preparation* (Figs. 10 and 11). The *restoration* refers to the material used in the reconstruction of the tooth.

Restorative Materials

The common dental restorations are as follows:

1. Amalgam—*silver fillings:* an alloy composed primarily of silver and tin mixed with mercury; used predominantly on posterior teeth and representing about 80 percent of all restorations.
2. Gold inlay: cast gold restoration made from an impression of the

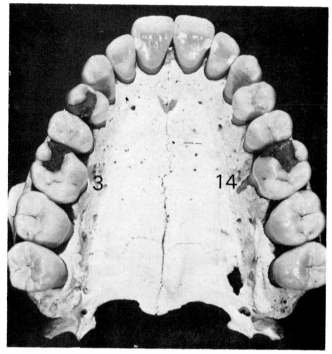

Figure 12. The maxilla or upper jaw showing a mesio-occlusal (MO) amalgam of the right first molar (3), a disto-occlusal (DO) amalgam of the right first premolar (5) and mesio-occlusal (MO) amalgam of the left first molar (14). Several silicate restorations are also present on the anterior teeth. See the postmortem chart of this jaw in Figure 14 below.

preparation and cemented in place; used on anterior and posterior teeth, gold in color, expensive.

3. Gold foil: a cohesive pure gold restoration wedged and molded into the preparation; generally used on small restorations involving anterior or posterior teeth, gold in color, expensive.

4. Crown—*cap:* a complete or partial extracoronal restoration which fits over the prepared tooth as a glove fits the hand; used on all teeth. A complete crown may be made of metal, acrylic resin or porcelain. The metal employed is usually gold, which may comprise the entire crown. Or, the crown may have superficial outer layers of porcelain or acrylic, partial or total, to cosmetically reproduce normal tooth color.

5. Silicate: an esthetic silica cement used on anterior teeth and appearing the same shade as surrounding tooth structure.

6. Acrylic: a plastic resin employed predominantly, like silicates, for restoration of anterior teeth; blends with surrounding tooth color.

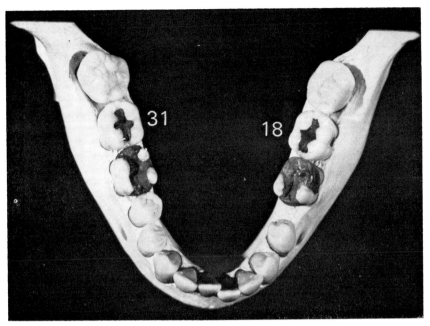

Figure 13. The mandible or lower jaw reveals single surface occlusal (O) amalgam restorations of the second molars (left, 18; right, 31). The left first molar (19) possesses a mesio-occluso-disto-bucco-lingual (MODBL) amalgam restoration. The right first molar (30) shows a mesio-occluso-distal amalgam with a lingual extension (MODL). Notice also that the left second premolar has been extracted in the remote past causing slight distal drift of the left first premolar. See the postmortem chart of this jaw in Figure 14.

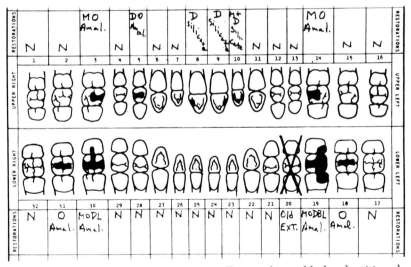

Figure 14. Postmortem dental chart of the maxillary and mandibular dentition shown in Figures 12 and 13. Note that normal teeth should be so designated (N).

7. Temporary cements: various white to gray to tan cements employed in incompleted restoration procedures.

Figures 12 and 13 represent dental arches from skeletal remains which portray various restorations involving numerous surfaces of the individual teeth. Figure 14 shows the corresponding postmortem dental chart of this case.

Tooth Loss and the Replacement of Teeth

The common causes of tooth loss are dental caries in the younger population (persons less than thirty years of age) and periodontal (gum) disease in the older population. Tooth loss presents both a functional and cosmetic detriment to the individual. The field of dentistry has several prosthetic devices to offer such individuals. A *prosthesis* is an artificial appliance utilized in the replacement or substitution of missing teeth. Such prosthetic appliances are either *fixed* or *removable* and are discussed below.

1. Fixed prosthesis—*a bridge:* a permanently attached appliance not easily removed by the patient or dentist. A bridge is a cemented device designed to span a gap in the dentition. The design usually consists of complete or partial crowns (retainers) of the abutment teeth (the natural teeth at either side of the gap) connected to a pontic section(s) substituting for the missing tooth or teeth responsible for the gap (Fig. 15). The metal involved is almost always gold; however, various porcelain or plastic coatings or facings may be employed for esthetic reasons. Figure 16 shows the components of a three-unit bridge on a dental model.

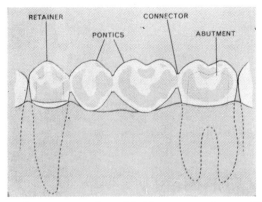

Figure 15. Diagrammatic representation of bridge nomenclature. The pontics represent the replaced teeth. The abutment teeth with retainer crowns support the pontics. The bridge is designated as a four-unit bridge. Courtesy of Morrey and Nelsen, *Dental Science Handbook.*

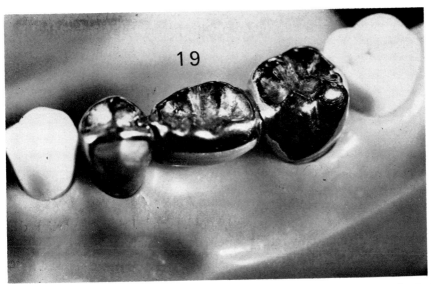

Figure 16. A three-unit bridge of the left lower jaw discloses teeth 18 and 20 (the second molar and second premolar, respectively) as abutments with 19 (first molar) representing the pontic. AFIP No. 73-1983-5.

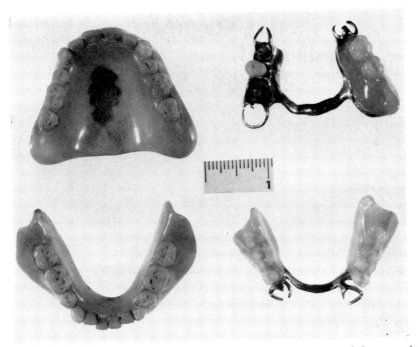

Figure 17. The difference between complete dentures (left) and partial dentures (right) is evident.

2. Removable prosthesis: (a) Complete or full denture—*false teeth:* composed of pink plastic base with permanently embedded teeth of porcelain or plastic; usually seen as a pair, i.e. upper and lower (Fig. 17). (b) Partial denture—*false teeth,* which in contrast to full dentures replace only a segment or segments of the natural dental arch; constructed of metallic and/or plastic base with teeth of plastic or porcelain; they attach to adjacent natural teeth by means of clasps and hooks (Fig. 17).

Radiographic Appearance of Dental Restorations or Procedures

The following statements apply to the radiographic appearance of dental restorations or procedures:

1. All dental metals (amalgam, gold, fixed bridges, partial denture framework) are markedly radiopaque when compared to tooth structure.

2. Silicate and acrylic restorations are radiolucent when compared to tooth structure.

3. Root canal cones are more radiopaque when contrasted with surrounding tooth structure.

FOR ADDITIONAL READING

Morrey, L. W., and Nelsen, R. J.: *Dental Science Handbook.* Washington, D.C., U.S. Government Printing Office, 1970.
Orban, B. J.: *Oral Histology and Embryology,* 4th ed. St. Louis, Mosby, 1957.

Chapter III

IDENTIFICATION OF UNKNOWN HUMAN REMAINS*

GENERAL COMMENTS

IDENTIFICATION of the unknown body is a medical, legal and humane responsibility which rests upon the shoulders of the forensic pathologist, coroner, dentist, law enforcement officer or any member of the team of forensic scientists called upon to evaluate data relevant to the identification. Identification of the deceased is necessary so that legal certification of death can be made. Such certification of death is necessary to consummate other legal matters such as insurance, wills, business interactions, remarriage of a spouse and lawsuits involving negligent parties. Religious interests of next of kin are served in instances where the absence of specific identification would result in the mass burial of multiple bodies of persons with different faiths. Furthermore, the establishment of identification following the mysterious disappearance and subsequent death of any given individual results in a termination of the agonizing emotional strain brought to bear on the loving, interested next of kin, engulfed in despair regarding the possible whereabouts of their beloved family member. This latter aspect has been recently brought to national attention by the inquiries and investigations demanded by families of armed forces personnel declared *missing in action* during the Viet Nam conflict. In converse fashion, the conclusion that remains are not those of a particular individual in question also represents a significant contribution by the identification expert. The latter situation is presently a common one regarding the hordes of runaway youngsters who fail to remain in contact with their families. Great relief is afforded concerned families who learn upon inquiry that the mass media report of an *unknown body found* does not represent the remains of their missing son or daughter.

The death certificate in the name of the identified deceased represents the legal proof of an individual's death. Without proof of death of a given individual, such as the unidentified body, a period of several years

---

* The core material of this chapter has appeared in an article previously published by the author in the *Journal of the American Dental Association*, 85:1324 (1972).

must elapse before an individual can be certified as legally deceased. In the state of Maryland, for example, a period of seven years must pass (with reasonable certainty that an individual is deceased) before a death certificate in the name of the deceased can be filed by the state medical examiner. Obviously, such an interval creates undue emotional and financial hardship for next of kin in any given case. The forensic identification expert derives gratification from the elimination of such hardship for others. Persons are born with an identity and deserve the right to die with an identity.

As the process of identification, or actually *reidentification*, applies to every unknown human body or parts thereof, it follows that identification will apply to cases involving each manner of death (see Chap. I). In addition to the above-discussed legal and moral reasons for identification, the homicide case conveys an added responsibility for identification personnel. In cases where the manner of death is homicide, identification of the remains provides the *corpus delicti* for subsequent legal proceedings and, furthermore, provides the core for subsequent police investigation surrounding the circumstances of death. This latter point is not to be dismissed lightly, since it is known that homicides usually involve family members or acquaintances. The establishment of the identity of the victim thereby facilitates the rapid accrual of important data pursuant to the entire police investigation and the eventual recovery of evidence relevant to the apprehension and conviction of the assailant. A known homicide involving an unidentified body generally results in an unsolved murder.

METHODS OF IDENTIFICATION OF THE UNKNOWN BODY

Various methods are employed in the establishment of identity of unknown remains. The reliability of each method varies depending upon the method used. Often the corroboration of identification by utilization of data gained from several of the less specific methods may elevate the probability of correct identification (to the acceptable standard of *reasonable medical certainty*) beyond that which could be obtained by either method alone. As will be explained, the method or methods used for identification are dictated by the postmortem condition of the body and/or the availability of antemortem data for comparison. An outline of identification methods is as follows:

1. The least reliable methods
    a. Visual recognition by next of kin or acquaintances
    b. Personal effects
2. The scientific methods
    a. Fingerprints

   b. Dental characteristics
   c. Skeletal characteristics
   d. Medical conditions
   e. Serology
   f. Hair
 3. Identification by exclusion

All of the methods of identification employ the basic process of *comparison*. This comparison involves known antemortem data versus established postmortem data. Successful comparison of these parameters, depending upon their specificity, equals identification. The specificity of the method used depends upon the frequency or occurrence, in the population at large, of the particular item or characteristic in question. For example, the finding of an appendectomy scar and absence of the appendix on postmortem examination may serve to narrow the field of possible identities but is in no way a specific finding due to its frequent occurrence in the population. On the other hand, one should keep in mind that the readily obtained facts regarding the absence of an appendix will immediately eliminate other persons being considered who are known not to have had an appendectomy. Similarly, the clothing of this same individual may not be specific, for usually there is nothing unique about a person's wearing apparel. In contrast, the uniqueness of the individual's fingerprints, specific for him alone, enables uncontestable declaration of positive identification.

The point to be stressed is that the fingerprint and the dental methods, in general terms, are the most specific and, hence, the most scientific methods of identification applicable to the human body. This is not to say that a particular skeletal or medical finding cannot also represent a very specific feature resulting in absolute identification. In a general sense, however, only the fingerprint or dental comparison results in absolute certainty of identification. The above-listed methods of identification are, in fact, scientific and most reliable since they represent physical characteristics with unmistakable, varying degrees of specificity inherent to the individual in question. The fingerprints and the teeth bear features which are specific characteristics of a single individual.

INTERRELATIONSHIP OF THE VARIOUS METHODS OF IDENTIFICATION
Least Reliable Methods of Identification
Visual Recognition by Relatives and Friends

This method represents the most frequent mode of identification if one considers all of the unknown bodies which are brought to a medical examiner's facility. Such *unidentified* bodies include numerous traffic accident victims and recent homicidal or natural deaths among individuals who have no immediate means of personal identification either by document or by the presence, at the scene of death, of persons who are familiar with the decedents. These cases generally involve recent deaths, and the bodies are well preserved with no effects of decomposition. In most of these cases, the investigating police soon after death are able to locate friends or next of kin. Such relatives can then establish identity by viewing the body and signing the necessary legal documents. The visual recognition of remains is limited to those cases where physical features of the body, especially the facial features, are not distorted by postmortem change or injury.

The rate at which a body decomposes after death is primarily dependent upon the environmental temperature. A body exposed to summer heat, especially when enclosed in a warm room, may not be outwardly recognizable after as short a time as twenty-four hours postmortem. In contrast, a body exposed to an outdoor winter climate in the middle Atlantic region may still be visually identifiable after a three- to four-month postmortem interval. It should be mentioned that even in winter conditions, a body exposed to carnivorous fauna may be so disfigured by rodents and larger animals that physical features may be completely obliterated long before any significant degree of decomposition has occurred (Fig. 18). The same is true of bodies in water subject to forage by marine life. To accept only visual recognition as the means of identification in such cases invites *mis-*

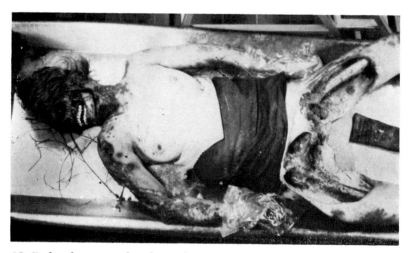

Figure 18. Body of a young female outdoors for three months in midwinter. The body exterior is well preserved except for the face and thigh-genital areas which disclose artefact due to wild animals. Identification was established by personal effects and dentition.

identification. There are numerous instances on record where visual identification of disfigured bodies has been proved erroneous by subsequent dental identification.[4-7]

Personal Effects (Clothing, Documents and Jewelry)

The mechanism of this mode of identification is at first sight self-explanatory. However, this method is *not* scientifically reliable due to the fact that clothing, documents and jewelry can be switched with criminal intent so that the deceased is, indeed, not the individual suggested by these effects. More commonly, these articles may be borrowed or even stolen. In general, clothing and personal effects decay at a slower rate than human soft tissues so that large portions of intact clothing, etc., may be relatively well preserved in the midst of skeletonized remains. Even in cases of marked incineration of the body, it is not unusual to find tattered, scorched clothing, a wallet, jewelry or other remnants which can provide essential putative clues to identification. Initialed rings and watches, keys, bracelets and belt buckles, etc., may render useful information toward a putative identification with more specific verification, by dental examination for example, following. Many articles are, however, mass-produced—common possessions to many and not distinctive. Even tarnished and rusted metallic objects can be chemically *pickled* to bare obscure features or engraved initials. Similarly, damaged and weathered documents can also be treated to reveal otherwise unrecognizable characteristics. The point of fact is that all potential personal items for identification should be saved for examination by the forensic identification laboratory. Prescription eyeglasses as well as contact lenses have served on occasion for identification. Clothing labels, laundry markings and the nature of the clothing may provide valuable clues as to social status, stature of the individual, place of purchase or laundry/cleaning facility.

This method is optimal when personal effects can be verified by other identification methods; however, in many instances personal belongings may serve as the only means of identity.

Scientific Methods of Identification

Fingerprints

Fingerprints are the most widely used scientific method of identification in this country today. The value of this method attests to the foresight of those who established the fingerprint system during the early 1900's. The FBI Fingerprint Division in Washington, D.C. currently has classified print files on approximately 84 million persons residing in the United States. The specificity of this method cannot be challenged, for there are no two sets of prints alike in their records. The disadvantages of the print system are two: (a) the all too frequent lack of an antemortem print record for comparison and (b) lack of sufficient postmortem fingerprint tissue for a determination of print classification. The latter shortcoming may be a result of injury, loss of soft tissue due to decomposition, or nonrecovery of the fingers. What many people do not realize is that when a list of possible identities for the deceased is submitted for comparison, only one half of the print region of a given finger is necessary for identification. This is of great importance in air crash victims where only portions of a single finger may be retrieved; however, when submitted with the passenger list, the identification can be established (assuming the availability of an antemortem print record). On the other hand, if one has an unknown body with no suspected identity, then a full complement of postmortem prints is necessary for the coding and record retrieval system to function.

The absence of an antemortem print record does not necessarily preclude possible identification because it may be possible to locate *latent* fingerprints on articles used by the deceased, such as hairbrushes, mirrors, glasses, doorknobs and other domestic articles. These latent prints can be compared with the postmortem prints of the deceased.

The uninitiated should not immediately dismiss the possibility of postmortem fingerprinting in cases of severe charring of the body or in instances of early decomposition or immersion of the body in water. Conflagration-induced contraction of the body musculature results in the *pugilistic or boxer's attitude* of the body which leads to *clenched fists.* Frequently, forced extension of the digits reveals protected, relatively intact pads of the fingers suitable for printing. Bodies immersed in water or showing early decomposition may have peeling of the skin of the hands; such hands should be gently disarticulated at the wrist joints and immediately forwarded to the fingerprint laboratory for analysis.

Dental Elements

One of the many ironic aspects of the natural world is that the human dentition, the site of prevalent, chronic breakdown in life, outlasts all other body tissues after death. The finding of intact dental elements in anthropological remains buried for centuries attests to this fact. In addition, dental restorations and prostheses are also extremely resistant to physical and chemical insult. The specificity of dental identification rests upon the innumerable combinations of restorations, prostheses, missing teeth and caries involving the 160 tooth surfaces visible on oral examination. In addition, the delineation of restoration morphology, root canal therapy and anatomic features of the teeth and paradontal tissues as revealed by roentgenographic examination further enhances the specificity of dental identification. The widespread utilization of dental care available in the civilized countries today represents the antemortem record *bank* for the dental identification comparison procedure. The improved maintenance of dental records and the rather ubiquitous employment of the dental X ray have served to amplify the specificity of the dental method as a scientific tool in identification.

In the United States, however, dental identification will never surpass the fingerprint method as the most reliable primary mode of identification of the unknown body. This is not necessarily true in other countries where fingerprint records are obtained only on criminals. Antemortem dental records, unlike fingerprints, are not easily obtained and recorded, are not centrally classified and are not readily retrievable for comparison. Furthermore, a list of possible identities must first be established in the procedure of dental identification so that antemortem records can be acquired from the attending dentist. An intact postmortem dentition may have numerous specific points of comparison; but if the antemortem record cannot be located no comparison is possible. Even with a list of possible identities regarding dental remains, days or months may elapse before the family of the deceased and, subsequently, the dentist who performed the work are located. In contrast, as mentioned earlier regarding fingerprints, a list of possible identities is not required for identification provided there is an antemortem record on file and a complete set of postmortem prints is obtained. Under these conditions identification by prints can be established in a matter of hours.

The paramount importance of dental identification is based upon the inherent deficits of the fingerprint method, namely, lack of an antemortem print record and/or absence of postmortem print tissue for comparison. It can be seen that dental identification advances gallantly to the fore in circumstances where both the visual and fingerprint methods are ineffectual, that is, following conflagration and/or extreme fragmentation, destruction or putrefaction of the body components. Indeed, the recovery of only a single tooth or jaw fragment may bear the degree of specificity necessary for positive identification.

For years, the armed forces have recognized the value of dental identification and have stressed the importance of up-to-date, accurate antemortem dental records. In civilian life, many companies employing high-risk accident-prone personnel, such as the airlines, maintain meticulous dental records including colored photographs of the dental structures. The author is aware of at least one professional football team that retains dental records as well as models of the team members.

Skeletal Remains

Given the proper conditions of environmental heat, moisture and insect activity, a body may be completely skeletonized within two months postmortem. Skeletal remains contain an abundance of information, which, when studied, can lead to reliable determination of race, sex, age and stature of the individual in life. In addition, an estimate of the interval between death and discovery of the remains can be made. Pathologic processes identified within the bones may provide evidence of disease or an old injury which can be compared with antemortem medical records or X rays. Occupational changes may also be reflected in the bones. In most instances, however, the skeleton lacks specificity regarding exact identity. Personal identity from skeletal examination is usually accomplished by means of the dentition. The value of skeletal examination is that it serves to greatly narrow the field of possible identities; hence, the method excludes large numbers of the population rather than identifies that single person whose skeleton it is. This method is commonly used in conjunction with the circumstances of disappearance and in corroboration of possible personal effects, etc., to establish a degree of certainty regarding the identification. Very often, skeletal examination focuses the identity within a most likely segment of the population, and antemortem dental records are searched in an effort to accomplish identification.

The totality of the skeletal remains, including bone fragments, should be retrieved from the scene of death and delivered to the medical examiner or pathologist responsible for the case. It should be remembered that various skeletal fragments can be reconstructed (using cement, wire, etc.) to reconstitute the skeletal features and delineate possible bone injuries that may be related to the cause of death. Even subtotal fragments of the long bones of the extremities may serve as indicators of the height of the subject during life. Even in the absence of the majority of the skeleton, microscopic examination of long bone fragments may serve as an indicator of chronologic age.[8]

The skull, primarily, and the long bones serve as indicators of race. Sex is most effectually determined upon examination of the pelvis, primarily, and the skull and long bones. In general terms, chronologic age of the skeleton is found by means of the dentition (see Chap. VIII), by consideration of the growth and development of the bones of the extremities and by age changes in the skull and of the symphysis pubis.

Although many forensic pathologists have received elementary exposure to basic techniques of skeletal identification, it is wise to have the services of a physical anthropologist available when necessary.

Medical (Autopsy and X rays) Facts

In addition to its prime importance in the establishment of cause and manner of death, the performance of the autopsy may also produce valuable data relevant to identification. Often a person's entire significant medical history can be suggested by the gross and microscopic examination of tissue obtained at autopsy. The comparison of these pathologic changes noted at postmortem examination with the known medical history of the suspected deceased serves to corroborate or dispute the putative identity. Individual specificity as to any abnormalities noted depends upon the diseases under consideration. Antemortem surgical procedures upon the body organs, recognized at autopsy, may serve to differentiate one body from the next and, if specific enough, can lead to identification. The body viscera also provide clues as to the age of the individual. Even in cases of severe charring of the body exterior, usually the internal organs are relatively unaffected and are quite suitable for study by the pathologist. General considerations regarding the forensic investigation of the burned body have been presented elsewhere by the author.[9]

The use of postmortem X-ray examination may disclose identifying characteristics of the skeletal structures, such as old fractures, arthritic changes, bone anomalies or even skull sinus outlines which, when compared with antemortem X rays, will lead to identification.

Clues such as body tattoos, moles or scars would apply to the autopsy, of course, as well as to visual recognition by friends.

Less specific findings from postmortem examination serve as useful data in that such information is utilized in corroboration with facts retrieved from the other methods employed.

Serology

The postmortem blood grouping of human tissues represents another source of scientific information which may be utilized in the comparison procedure. Due to the relative frequencies of the various ABO, MN and RH blood groupings, this method by itself is not specific; however, it serves to corroborate or reinforce other modes of identification. A known postmortem blood grouping for an individual serves to narrow the range of possible identities. The inability to obtain whole blood postmortem does not eliminate the use of serology in identification since even fragments of congested tissues, such as lung, liver or skeletal muscle can be utilized for blood group determination. Even in putrefied bodies with advanced decomposition, blood group antigens may still be detectable for serologic studies. The bone marrow in skeletal remains may still retain serologically detectable antigens.

Hair

The microscopic examination of body hair enables a classification to be made as to the race of an individual. Various differences between human and nonhuman hair can also be determined. The scalp hair, especially, decays at a slower rate than the more vulnerable soft body tissues upon decomposition, and tufts of hair often may be found adjacent to the skull in skeletonized remains. The hair can thus be utilized to substantiate the racial determination suggested by the skeleton. The color of the hair, the presence of hair dyes and the possible existence of scalp disease can also be detected.

Identification by Exclusion

This phenomenon refers to the establishment of identity based upon a comparison of the postmortem data of the deceased with known antemortem data pertaining to others. This is best illustrated by the following example:

> A chartered airliner crashes killing all twenty persons aboard. All occupants are burned beyond recognition. The passenger-crew manifest lists nineteen males and a female stewardess. The mere finding of female sex organs within a given body on postmortem examination establishes the identity of this body as that of the known stewardess. There is nothing specific pertaining to the female remains; however, by exclusion, the body must be that of the stewardess.

Identification by exclusion would also apply to the identification of infant or child remains if it is known that an infant or child was definitely the sole such occupant of a burning dwelling, for example. Another example of exclusion would be the identification of several charred children in an air crash setting, wherein they were the only children on board and were so dissimilar in age that skeletal or dental features enabled identification based upon age only as a differential feature. The basis for identification in such instances consists of the correlation of established antemortem facts with nonspecific postmortem data; however, exclusionary information provides positive identification.

SUMMARY OF THE GENERAL IDENTIFICATION FORMAT

All the above methods may be utilized in various combinations whenever necessary for identification of unknown human remains. The visual and fingerprints methods are the simplest to employ. If these methods cannot be utilized or are fruitless, then the dental method becomes of the utmost importance. The fingerprint and the dental methods are the most scientifically reliable and also the most specific. The methods which may bear lesser degrees of specificity (medical history, personal effects, skeletal features, serology, hair), nevertheless, are valuable assets in the identification format. The data derived from these methods is pooled to enable as many points of comparison as possible to be used in elevating the degree of credibility regarding a particular identification. Identification is accomplished by means of comparisons. Obviously, the greater the number of criteria for comparison, the more reliable is the comparison. The following cases demonstrate the interaction of the various methods of identification and the process of data collection:

An unidentified decomposed female body is recovered in an isolated wooded area. The following facts are established regarding the identity of the remains:

1. Considering the local climate and environmental conditions wherein the body is found, the interval since death is estimated at two to four weeks. Visual identification is impossible due to putrefactive changes.

2. An appendectomy scar and surgically absent appendix serve as a corroborative feature in identification but alone are not of major value due to the high occurrence of this condition in the population (medical facts).

3. Aging of the organs indicates that the deceased was about thirty to forty years of age (medical fact). The pubic symphysis segment of the pelvis also suggests the age to be thirty to forty years (skeletal remains).

4. Fingerprints are obtained from the remains; however, there are no antemortem print records for comparison on file with the local police or the central FBI laboratories (fingerprints).

5. Brown hair samples recovered from the remains are determined to be of the caucasoid race (hair).

6. The clothing is nondescript and reveals no laundry marks or other specific characteristics. There is an absence of distinctive jewelry or documents (personal effects).

7. The blood type is group O. This particular blood type is too frequent to be of specific value but can be used to exclude the deceased from other considered identities with a different blood type (serology).

8. The postmortem dental examination reveals that numerous amalgam restorations and endodontic treatment have been performed on a maxillary second molar. These dental findings represent the most specific identifying characteristics of the remains. The remaining problem is to arrive at a proposed (putative) identity of the deceased and then locate any antemortem dental records (dental elements).

9. The missing persons bureau is contacted regarding a possible report on a thirty- to forty-year-old white female of the estimated body height, weight, hair color and clothing characteristics, etc. Three names are forwarded from their files for consideration. Interrogation of the families of these three individuals reveals that one was totally edentulous but had had a previous appendectomy. The second name proposed had a previous radical mastectomy for breast cancer, a condition not noted at autopsy, thus eliminating this person from consideration. The third individual's record is obtained from the family dentist, and a perfect dental comparison is made including a 2mm overfill of the mesiobuccal root of the maxillary second molar.

Identification in this case was accomplished upon analysis of the data retrieved from a thorough forensic postmortem examination. The dental examination represented the only means whereby conclusive identification could be achieved.

A final case is presented to emphasize the importance of total postmortem data collection and the role of summation of probability to establish a reasonably certain identification. The case also emphasizes the need for complete communication and cooperation between the law enforcement agency and the medical examiner facility:

A totally charred body, a victim of homicide, was recovered from a burning vehicle parked on an isolated country road. Scorched remnants of clothing disclosed that the victim was wearing two undershirts (among more usual attire), and scalp hair remnants were identified as Negroid in origin. The skull, despite its charred condition, enabled an age estimate to be established for the deceased at thirty to thirty-five years. The owner of the burned vehicle (J.W.), as established through license plate registration, was found to be missing and the initial impression was that the body in question was that of the thirty-plus-year-old Negro vehicle owner. Antemortem dental records and X rays pertaining to the latter failed to compare with the postmortem dental findings and X rays of the victim. Subsequent police investigation of the whereabouts of the vehicle owner produced information indicating that the body might be that of a close friend (J.G.), an individual with whom J.W. was in company several hours prior to discovery of the burning vehicle. The clothing remnants recovered from the body were shown to the mother of J.G., and she identified the print pattern on a shirt as being the shirt her son wore the evening preceding the fire; and further, she stated that her son characteristically wore two undershirts as he was always cold. In efforts to substantiate the identification as being that of J.G., an exhaustive effort to locate all antemortem medical and dental records for this individual was made. J.G.'s medical data revealed his height as five feet, ten inches, consistent with the estimated height of the deceased as derived from the intact humerus of the burned body. In addition, a curvature of the spine noted on an antemortem chest X ray report was also a finding of the postmortem examination. The only antemortem dental record consisted of a notation that teeth 18 and 31 were extracted. No dental X rays or charts were ever located. The absence of these two teeth on the victim was therefore consistent with the dental records for J.G.; however, the dental comparison for J.G. was by means specific for him alone. There was no record of an antemortem blood type to compare with the postmortem serologic data. Further search of the medical records disclosed that J.G. had a varicocele (an abnormality of the left scrotum) noted on prior physical examination several years earlier. Despite the charred condition of the body the presence of a left scrotal varicocele was noted upon dissection.

Again, identification of the above case resulted from the combination of facts derived from the circumstances of death, clothing, skeletal findings and hair, and the dental and medical examinations. The disclosure of a rare and unusual medical finding (varicocele) in conjunction with the accumulated data established the personal identification.

Chapter IV

THE UTILIZATION OF DENTAL METHODS FOR THE IDENTIFICATION OF AIRCRAFT ACCIDENT FATALITIES*

INTRODUCTION

THE AUTHOR THINKS it can be safely stated that the aircraft accident results in greater destruction upon the human body as compared to other commonly occurring disasters. With this point in mind, it is important to survey the role of dental methods in the identification of such victims. In addition to the moral, emotional and legal ramifications incumbent to the identification of any unknown body, the air crash setting brings forth several other cogent reasons for the establishment of victim identification. From the standpoint of the aeronautical engineer, the air safety specialist, the air accident investigation team and the aerospace or forensic pathologist, victim identification provides important data which may lead to improvement of the man-machine relationship as it applies to aircraft. The primary goal of the multidisciplinary approach to the air accident is the prevention of future accidents. Inherent in this objective are the answers to why the survivors lived and why and by what means the victims died. The identification of air accident victims enables an assessment to be made regarding known seating locations and crash scene data to allow reconstruction of crash mechanics and the mechanism of injury patterns. The adequacy of existing escape exits in fallen aircraft can be evaluated, for example. In addition, the identification of particular crew members enables the pathologist to assess the role that natural disease may have exercised in any given accident. As an example, a question may arise as to whether disease-induced incapacitation of the pilot may have resulted in the accident. The pathologist may discover a diseased heart, but is it from the pilot or whom?

---

* The core material of this chapter has appeared in an article previously published by the author in the *Journal of Forensic Sciences*, 18:356 (1973).

THE AIR CRASH AS A DISASTER

In terms of feasibility of identification of remains, an advantage and a disadvantage apply to the aircraft accident as compared to other mass disasters, such as floods, fires, explosions in public buildings, mine disasters and other mass-transportation accidents. The advantage concomitant to the air disaster is that a passenger-crew manifest is usually available, a fact which greatly narrows the probable population segment involved, thus allowing the identification team to concentrate upon a comparison between postmortem data on a set of *unknowns* with a determined closed set of *known* antemortem data. Such a list of putative identities is, of course, essential for the process of dental identification because the antemortem record for comparison must be retrieved from an attending dentist. In other forms of mass disaster, however, in which a previously established list of possible identities is unavailable, almost endless possibilities of identity exists, which necessitate prolonged investigations involving extreme amounts of time and effort.

Several contrasts also exist upon comparing the civilian air crash with a corresponding military air accident. The dental identification of military air crash victims is more readily proven than that of the civilian accident victims. The reason for this is that the antemortem dental records of military personnel are more rapidly located and are generally accurate and recent in origin. In addition, the military accident rarely involves the large number of victims as is common with the commercial air carrier disaster. The presence of fire-resistant metallic ID tags and fire-resistant flight clothing among military personnel also allows for rapid establishment of a putative identity for possible dental confirmation.

The disadvantage regarding identification in an air crash setting centers upon the mutilating high-impact forces common to such accidents and the frequent intensity and duration of subsequent conflagration. Both of these aspects inherent to the air crash lead to loss of physical features, which frequently precludes the use of the visual and fingerprint methods of identification and may even jeopardize the efficacy of the dental method.

When dealing with identification in aircraft disasters, the identification team faces a conflicting situation. On the one hand, cognizant of the medical, legal and emotional aspects involved, the preference would be to utilize the most scientifically specific modes of identification—the fingerprint or dental method. On the other hand, the team must not lose sight of the practical facets of the total situation. In the aftermath of a plane crash, when faced with seventy or one hundred (or more) bodies, many of whom may be identified by clothing, documents, jewelry and personal belongings, the realm of practicality must prevail; and these less reliable methods may have to suffice as modes of identification. This is not to say that, with time and effort, dental identification of many of these victims could not be accomplished. Given the personnel and the time, dental identification could be achieved, but this represents the ideal situation and not the more commonly encountered situation in which time and skilled personnel are in short supply. This point must be kept in mind when interpreting numerical data regarding the role of dental identification in air crashes. A statement that dental features were responsible for the identification of 15 percent of a given number of victims often reflects the outcome of what was practical as opposed to what was ideal. This must not necessarily be interpreted to mean that only 15 percent of the victims could be identified by dental means. The correct interpretation is that 15 percent were easily recognized by this means. An important point that surfaces from the foregoing discussion is that a pre-established dental disaster squad (DDS), namely, an organized team of several dentists, can more effectively implement dental identification among disaster victims and thereby more nearly approach the ideal situation.

The statistical significance of dental identification in any particular air crash (or mass disaster) is inversely related to the workability of the visual, fingerprint and personal effects methods. In instances in which there is relative absence of mutilating injuries and conflagration, these nondental methods will inevitably rank as the primary modes of identification. This, of course, assumes that next of kin are available for interrogation and for recognition of remains and that antemortem fingerprint records are available. These assumptions do not usually hold in instances of international carriers disasters, in which relatives are not nearby nor are fingerprint records of citizens maintained by the country in question. It is the very problem of dental identification in international disasters that has prompted the Federation Dentaire Internationale to establish a universal dental numbering system that enables easy telegraphic transmission of dental records between countries.

The effectiveness of dental identification in any particular instance is directly related to the recovery of dental remains (all, none or partial), the retrieval of antemortem records and the recency and accuracy of these records. A breakdown in recency or accuracy of records may lead to disturbing inconsistencies and incompatibilities. The lack of available antemortem records leaves one with a relative's recollection regarding the teeth of the victim or, at best, the memory of the attending dentist.

DENTAL IDENTIFICATION IN AIRCRAFT ACCIDENTS

Table III is a collation of statistical data relating to the use of dental identification in aircraft accident fatalities. These figures represent international experience, since British,[10, 16, 18, 23] New Zealand,[15] Scandinavian,[12] South African,[20] Canadian[21] and American[11, 13, 14, 17, 19, 22] identification data are cited. Twenty-two accidents, involving 1,080 fatalities, are represented. The number and percentage of victims identified solely by dental means and with the assistance of dental examination are presented in columns A and B, respectively. The summation of data indicates that dental examination alone or in conjunction with other methods was responsible for the identification of 40 percent of all fatalities. Dental examination alone provided the identification of 32.8 percent of the victims.

This overall figure of 32.8 percent represents a mean percentage including much variability. Examining the data more closely, one sees the following extremes represented: Luntz and Luntz,[22] Harmeling, et al.[17] and Haines[23] presented data revealing that 89 percent, 75 percent and 74 percent of the victims, respectively, were identified by their teeth. At the opposite end of the spectrum, Stevens and Tarlton,[16] Teare[10] and Blair[15] reported 10, 11 and 13 percent, respectively. The explanation of such variability depends upon the many factors in operation at the time of the accident. Obviously, not all air accidents present the same circumstances, since the degree of mutilation and conflagration varies. As has been mentioned earlier, the condition of the victims also varies with regard to the efficacy

TABLE III

DENTAL IDENTIFICATIONS IN AIRCRAFT ACCIDENT FATALITIES

Author(s) or Accidents	Number of Accidents	Number of Fatalities	A. Identification By Dentition Only No.	%	B. Identification Assisted By Dentition No.	%
Teare,[10] 1951	1	28	3	11	—	—
Honolulu, Hawaii,[11] 1962	1	27	14	52	—	—
Kieser-Nielsen,[12] 1963	1	42	10	24	18	43
Salley, et al.,[13] 1963	2	127	62	49	—	—
Fisher,[14] 1963	1	81	3	4	13	16
Blair,[15] 1964	1	23	3	13	10	43
Stevens and Tarlton,[16] 1966	8	218	21	10	—	—
Harmeling, et al.,[17] 1966	1	57	43	75	—	—
Haines,[18] 1967	1	72	34	47	6	8
Boone County, Ky.,[19] 1967	1	67	19	28	—	—
Van Wyk, et al.,[20] 1969	1	123	6	5	25	20
Petersen and Kogon,[21] 1971	1	109	53	49	—	—
Luntz and Luntz,[22] 1972	1	28	25	89	—	—
Haines,[23] 1972	1	78	58	74	—	—
	22	1,080	354	32.8	72	7.2

and practicality of application of the various methods employed in general identification. The mere availability and utilization of a dentist or team of dentists may also be reflected in these data.

Luntz and Luntz[22] reported twenty-five of twenty-eight burned victims identified by the dentition within seventy-two hours after the accident. The success of these authors attests to the efficiency of a local dental disaster squad. This team of dentists was completely prepared to handle such a disaster. The personnel, necessary equipment for examination, and liaison with the local police, medical examiner's office and legal authorities had been established months beforehand. Harmeling, et al.[17] had a team of four dentists operating in the dental identification of 75 percent of the fifty-seven victims of the 1965 Cincinnati air crash. Both this accident and the Luntz crash in Connecticut involved severe conflagration, and the work of these dental teams portrays what can reasonably be expected from the mandatory utilization of dental identification when other methods of identification are useless. The Canadian Woodbridge air disaster, discussed later in this chapter, is another example of the results obtained when the team approach is utilized. These accounts should serve as models for similar dental teams and should be prepared in advance to assist in the event of any mass disaster. It is hoped that the dental schools of the world will serve as the centers for the establishment of such teams, each assisting within its area of legal jurisdiction under the auspices of the responsible medical examiner, coroner or law enforcement system. Currently, in the United States, the American Society of Forensic Odontology is establishing a list of dental practitioners willing to participate in dental identification cases arising in their locality.

Salley, et al.[13] reported on two air disaster experiences within a two-year period, each involving extreme burning of victims, wherein results were contrasting. The first crash wreckage burned for ten hours before the bodies could be extracted, making dental examination possible on only seventeen of the fifty remains. Of these seventeen cases, however, these workers were able to identify thirteen by teeth alone. In the second crash, which burned for six and one-half hours prior to body recovery, dental examinations were performed on seventy-six of the seventy-seven fatalities, and dental identification was established on forty-nine (64%).

Haines[18] reported on the Stockport, England air disaster, in which the majority of remains were severely damaged by fire. In no instance were the jaws sufficiently damaged to prevent employment of dental identification. Thirty-four of the seventy-two victims (47%) were identified by dentition alone, including eighteen persons who possessed full dentures. An addi-

tional six identifications initially established by other methods were subsequently verified by dental examination. In two cases of supposed visual
identification of remains, these were proved to be in error by the dental
examination.

Haines[23] produced another fine effort in his dental identification work
in the Rijeka air disaster. The severe post-crash conflagration resulted in
seventy-eight charred fatalities. Haines and his team produced fifty-eight
(74%) identifications based upon dentition alone, including eight cases by
dental exclusion. Fourteen bodies were identified by nondental methods.
Five bodies remained unidentified, necessitating mass burial of these individuals. Each of the five unidentified bodies possessed full dentures; however, further points of individual specificity could not be obtained. The
latter fact points out the necessity for the characterization of individual
dentures by the incorporation of an identifying name or number in the
denture manufacture process (see Chap. VII).

One must not become so enmeshed in such a statistical scorecard that one
forgets that the overall value of dental identification rests not only on
those cases in which identification solely by teeth is effected but also upon
those in which the dental examination was utilized to assist the credibility
of other methods of identification and thus played a contributory role.
Blair[15] identified by teeth alone three of twenty-three victims (13%) of the
Kaimai, New Zealand crash, but the dentition assisted the identification of
ten more victims; thus, the dental examination was of value in more than
one half of the total identifications. Blair states that the dental evidence
was, on the whole, the most valuable mode of identification despite the
fact that the dentition of five of the nineteen recovered bodies was completely lost. Blair encountered problems with melted dentures and appall-
ingly poor antemortem dental records. He also described the heat-induced
loss of anterior silicate and acrylic restorations with the affected teeth presenting surfaces that could be mistaken for carious lesions. In addition,
the vaporization and surfacing of mercury droplets from amalgam restorations were noted to discolor adjacent gold inlays, thus imparting to the
latter the coloration of amalgam. Similarly, Keiser-Nielsen[12] reported a
Scandinavian airline crash in Ankara, Turkey in which forty-two passengers died. Dental evidence played an important role in twenty-eight
identifications (66%), although the dental method alone accounted for ten
fatalities only. Twenty-one of these twenty-eight persons were identified
exclusively or primarily by the dentition; three children were identified by
age determination based upon their dentition; in four victims identification by the teeth assisted other methods. In three of the forty-two deaths,
no dental remains were located; nine victims had examinable dental re-

mains, but no antemortem records existed. Dental identification of the 123 Windhoek, South Africa air crash victims, as reported by Van Wyk, et al.,[20] accounted for only 5 percent of the total number of bodies, but the dental method assisted in an additional 20 percent of the identifications. In the 1963 Elkton, Maryland accident, Fisher,[14] although utilizing fingerprint identification primarily, found that 20 percent of the total identification of eighty-one victims were facilitated to varying degrees by dental examination.

The account by Stevens and Tarlton[16] of 218 fatalities resulting from eight air accidents provides some insight into the relative frequencies, in their experience, of the different modes of identification. They reported that dental identification was effective in 10 percent of these fatalities. By comparison, documents (25%), jewelry (20%), clothing (16%) and medical records (12%) accounted for the majority of the identifications. The extent to which dentists or dental methods were utilized is not indicated in the article.

It is important to realize that what is considered acceptable evidence of positive identification rests with the authorities governing the investigation of the air accident and depends upon the presence or absence of certain circumstances surrounding the incident. Certainly, in any accident occurring as a result of criminal activity such as skyjacking, terrorism or extortion plots, it is mandatory that an attempt be made to identify all bodies conclusively by either the fingerprint or the dental method. One must keep in mind that personal effects and clothing may be unreliable, because such items may be borrowed, stolen or switched with criminal intent.

An earlier article by Stevens and Tarlton[24] reveals the interplay of various methods of identification as applied to air crashes. They reported on four aircraft accidents (the data from three of these were included in their later article[16]) involving 116 fatalities. Accident 1 involved extensive mutilation but only minimal effects of conflagration, so that personal effects (clothing, documents, jewelry) accounted for 89 percent of the identifications. Dental identification accounted for 8 percent of the victims. The relative absence of fire, thus permitting identification by personal effects in this accident, was fortunate, as thirty-four of the thirty-nine persons aboard were male children aged twelve to fourteen years. Efficient dental identification in mass disasters involving large numbers of young children of approximately the same age is extremely difficult.[25] This especially pertains to a fluoride-treated population, in which decay and restorations are few. Fingerprint identification is also of no value in accidents involving children because of the lack of preexisting records. Ashley[26] reports of the identification, through estimation of dental age, of sixteen children involved in an air accident. The 1969 London air disaster, primarily involving Asian nationals, included sixteen passengers less than sixteen years of age. The paucity of restorations and lack of readily available antemortem records, even if existing, necessitated the use of dental age estimation as the primary means of identification. Ashley established estimations of chronologic age as derived from dental development and compared these estimations with the known age and sex of the children as provided on the passenger manifest. His method of dental age derivation initially included an approximation of age on the basis of the erupted dentition. Selected teeth were then removed and examined to more accurately delineate the dental age from the degree of crown and root development. Using the tables of Massler-Schour (see Chap. VIII), the stages of crown and root development enabled a more exact estimation of dental age. The dental age as determined (in conjunction with sex as determined by the pathologist) was then matched with the known age and sex provided in the passenger list.

Air crashes 3 and 4 reported by Stevens and Tarlton[24] involved substantial post-crash fires. Dental identification was effective in 18 and 21 percent, respectively, among fifteen and twenty-six victims. In three of their four reported accidents, they stated that the dental method was quantitatively of greater value in identification than a complete medical examination (autopsy and roentgenologic).

The recently formed Canadian Society of Forensic Odontology was summoned by local authorities and played a major role in the identification of 109 victims of the Woodbridge, Canada DC-8 crash in July 1970.[21] The task of identifying these dismembered victims necessitated the efforts of twelve dentists at one time or another over a sixteen-day period. The immense challenge facing these workers consisted of the identification of 134 separate jaw specimens and 37 denture fragments contained within 800 bags of remains retrieved from the accident site. These figures are presented to impress the reader with the fact that one is faced with the prospect of mass air disasters involving aircraft of still greater size and capacity. Dental identification in the event of such an accident would almost demand an organized team of experts. Perhaps some thought should be given to the establishment of government-funded squads of dental experts who would be able to assist at disaster sites, much as the FBI Fingerprint Team does today in the United States.

The Woodbridge, Canada team was able to retrieve antemortem dental records of 67 of the 109 victims. Primary identification by teeth was made in 53 (49%) of the 109 victims. The fifty-three identifications represented 60 percent of all the identifications effected in that disaster. Dental identification was made in 72 percent of the cases in which useful antemortem records were available. Age estimation based on dentition proved to be of valuable assistance in the eventual identification of infants, children and young adults. The account of the Woodbridge disaster[21] should be studied by those interested in the field of mass-disaster identification, since it describes in detail the thorough investigation and presents the use of 35mm slide photography of dental specimens in the comparison procedure.

While it is true that the purpose of this chapter is to survey and emphasize the role of dental identification in the air crash setting, the author wishes to repeat that one must not lose sight of the overall relationship between forensic dentistry and the other methods of identification (Chap. III). What the reader must not fail to realize is that, when circumstances permit, the use of fingerprint identification ranks superior in every respect to dental identification. This statement applies primarily to the United States and its citizens, because other countries do not maintain such extensive fingerprint files of their populations. For this reason fingerprint identification is conspicuously absent from the foregoing accounts of foreign accident identification investigations. The lack of fingerprint files in other countries also attests to the even greater need for dental identification personnel in these countries. J. K. Mason, the internationally known British aviation pathologist, has stated that dental identification currently occupies a primary role in the identification of British air disaster victims.[27]

Due to the availability of the FBI fingerprint identification agency in this country (Chap. III), it is impractical to initially apply dental identification procedures to every body recovered from an air accident. The crash situation must be surveyed, and the potential need for dental methods should be evaluated. The fingerprint method should immediately be used on suitable bodies, and the dental examiners should then concentrate on those cases in which the fingerprint method is unworkable. In the ideal situation, if time and personnel permit, dental identification can substantiate those identifications established on the basis of personal effects. This represents a rational approach to the matter and is the course commonly followed in air crashes occurring in the United States. The identification data of the 1963 Elkton, Maryland crash handled by Fisher[14] exemplifies this. Of eighty-one victims, fifty-three were identified by fingerprints and three were identified by teeth alone; the teeth assisted in thirteen other identifications. Other accidents in the continental United States involving United States nationals reveal similar data[28-32] (see Table IV).

As stated in Chapter III, in the United States, under circumstances where postmortem tissue is available for fingerprinting and an antemortem record exists for comparison, dental identification will never surpass the

TABLE IV

UTILIZATION OF FINGERPRINT IDENTIFICATION IN CONTINENTAL
U.S. AIR ACCIDENT FATALITIES

Accident	No. Victims	Fingerprint Identification	Other Identification
Boston, Mass.			
Electra,[28] 1960	61	All identified by fingerprints, acquaintances, or personal effects	
Lake Tahoe, Nev.			
Constellation,[29] 1964	85	79	2 dental
Portland, Ore.			
DC-9,[30] 1966	18	5	10 dental and personal effects
Urbana, Ohio			
Midair,[31] 1967	25	18	7 dental and/or autopsy
Blossburg, Pa.			
BAC-111,[32] 1967	34	26	4 dental
Elkton, Md.			
Boeing 707,[14] 1963	81	53	16 dental and/or other methods

fingerprint method as the primary mode of identification. The fingerprint identification is more quickly and easily performed, and the antemortem records for comparison are centrally coded and classified. Fingerprint identification can be established in a matter of hours, if necessary. The process of dental identification does not possess these attributes. The dental postmortem examination is time-consuming; the acquisition of antemortem dental records is a lengthy, frustrating experience necessitating direct vocal and/or mail communication with the attending dentists. The use of airline clerks has proved unsatisfactory.[13, 21] The actual dental comparison, once both antemortem and postmortem data are in hand, is again a tedious and time-consuming procedure.

The loss of fingerprint tissue applies not only to cases of conflagration but also to instances of skeletonization of remains. The application of dental identification to skeletal remains and the relative indestructibility of the dentition and dental restorations are revealed by the recent experience of Sopher and Angel.[33] These authors had occasion to identify the remains of seventeen military personnel who died in an air crash of a World War II military transport. The remains were found in the jungle highlands of New Guinea twenty-seven years after the loss of the aircraft. Dental remains were recovered from twelve of the seventeen victims, and subsequent conclusive dental identification was effected in these twelve persons by virtue of available, accurate antemortem military dental records.

Chapter V

BASIC CONCEPTS OF DENTAL IDENTIFICATION: THE ANTEMORTEM DATA

THE VALIDITY OF DENTAL IDENTIFICATION

THE USE OF THE TEETH as a means of identification of the unknown body is based on the same principle that is common to the other methods of identification, namely, the principle of *comparison*. The fact that finger-prints and the dentition represent rather permanent signatures quite unique for the individual in question is the reason why these physical characteristics stand alone as being the most scientifically reliable methods of identification. A reliable method of identification must embody certain criteria to allow valid application to the principle of comparison. These criteria include

1. a medium which possesses multiple, permanent, measurable or observable points of specificity so that relative individuality of the medium exists;
2. previous accurate registration of the characteristics of individuality (the antemortem data) that must be available for comparison with any subsequently retrieved data (the postmortem data); and
3. a medium, complete with its contained features of specificity, that must be resistant to destructive forces so that it persists as a pillar of individuality in the absence of other identifying features.

The criteria of individuality, previous registration and relative indestructibility are characteristics especially applicable to the dentition and are responsible for the importance of the dental structures as a scientific tool in identification. The process of dental identification involves a comparison between the antemortem registration of dental features as noted in dental records and the dental data retrieved upon postmortem examination of the remains. Any breakdown in the criteria mentioned above may jeopardize or nullify the reliability of the comparison process.

Each of the above-mentioned criteria as applied to the human dentition will be discussed in turn below.

Individuality of the Dentition

The individuality or specificity of the dentition is based upon the multiple points of comparison inherent in a variable combination of events which alter the status of a given set of thirty-two teeth, each comprising five anatomic surfaces. Such events include (1) hereditary, congenital or developmental alterations; (2) acquired natural or traumatic alterations; (3) the presence or absence in multiple combinations of one, many or most of the thirty-two units; and (4) the combinations and permutations in the variable construction, constitution and morphology of a various array of restorative procedures, materials and prosthetic devices employed by the dental profession. In addition, the innumerable features of the dental and jaw structures as revealed by the roentgenogram further enhance the criterion of individuality. In instances where chronologic age exercises a role in the identification, the added dimension of time and its effect on the teeth is introduced as a measurable criterion.

Very concisely, the presence of 160 available dental surfaces (32 teeth times 5 surfaces) subject to alteration by decay and restoration, the latter process including numerous materials of varying shape and size, as well as the innumerable combinations of one or more missing teeth at variable locations impart uniqueness or specificity to the dental medium.

Indeed, a basic premise of dental identification is that no two mouths are identical. Theoretically, this may represent a true statement; however, in actuality the reliability of this statement depends upon the number of points of specificity available for the comparison between the antemortem and the postmortem data in any particular case. The greater the number of quantitative and qualitative points of comparison, the more reliable is the comparison and the more nearly one approaches this axiom. Computer models have shown that there are more than 2.5 billion possibilities in charting the human mouth.[34] Much effort is currently being expended in evaluating the efficacy of computerized dental charts as a means of classifying mass identification data.

Previous Registration

The second criterion, that of previous registration, is dependent upon the existence, retrievability and quality of the antemortem dental records as maintained by an attending dentist of the putative deceased. To be sure, the ubiquitous availability of mass dental care in the more advanced societies of the modern world in conjunction with the maintenance of dental records including dental X rays has served to greatly enhance the use of the teeth and oral structures as a means of identification. It is ironic, however, in the face of this statement, that the failure to satisfy the criterion of accurate previous registration is all too often responsible for the inability to identify remains which are noted to contain numerous dental points of specificity. This criterion may not be satisfied due to absent, poor or inaccurate records as maintained by a known attending dentist[35, 36] or because of the inability to locate the dentist responsible for the work in question. The latter situation results when one cannot arrive at a proposed (putative) identity of the deceased to enable family members to provide a dentist's record. In other instances, of course, the family may not know of the attending dentist.

The establishment of a proposed or putative identity of the remains is essential for the process of dental identification. This constitutes a major disadvantage in the method of dental comparison, and rectification of this problem is the precise objective of mass computerization of dental records. Such computerization would establish a record retrieval system similar to the current concepts in operation for fingerprint identification. The author's mention of computer efforts in relation to dental records does not necessarily indicate that he feels the endeavor can be successful. In theory, the system is quite sound. In application, however, the method incorporates vast problems in the maintenance of up-to-date records and requires the complete cooperation of a very busy group of people, the dental practitioners. The author thinks the concept is possible within limited populations but doubts its success when applied to the population at large.

The antemortem dental data bank available for comparison with the postmortem examination data rests within the records of the attending dentist. Such records consist of the patient's dental chart, dental X rays and, in some instances, stone casts or models made from impressions of the dentition. These items are elucidated later in this chapter.

The weakest and least reliable source of antemortem data is the recollection by family members of dental traits of the deceased. Certain noticed dental peculiarities (gaps between teeth, gold crowns, fractured teeth) may stand the test of comparison and, if specific, may enable an identification to be established. Such recollections are frequently erroneous[35] or valueless but, on the other hand, may provide information which can be pooled with other identification data to elevate the probability of correct identification. Personal photographs, upon magnification or enlargement, also provide information regarding characteristics of the anterior dentition.

Of historical interest, before the existence of patient dental records, cases are cited of personal identification based upon the mere presence or absence of teeth, the general condition of the teeth, peculiar alignment of the dentition as well as the presence of restorations or dentures. Paul Revere, the *Minute Man* dentist, utilized dental features in the recognition of the remains of Doctor Joseph Warren, a patriot killed at Bunker Hill.[37] The exhumed body of John Wilkes Booth, Lincoln's assassin, was identified by a gold-plugged tooth on the right side of his jaw.[38]

Indestructibility of the Dentition

The third criterion, that of indestructibility, is especially applicable to dental structures and the metallic agents used in restorations and prostheses. The preservation of intact teeth in anthropological remains buried for centuries attests to this fact. The enamel of tooth structure is one of the hardest minerals found in the natural world and is the hardest calcified substance in the body. The teeth, upon exposure to postmortem influences, outlast all other body tissues. Dental metals are also extremely resistant to destructive physical and chemical forces.

The direct effects of fire and associated heat constitute a much greater threat to the integrity of the teeth and dental restorations than do the processes of postmortem putrefaction. In view of this statement further discussion is in order. In household conflagrations the dentition is generally intact and very frequently represents the only means of identification. In contrast, high-intensity fires, as noted in chemical and fuel-fed industrial and aircraft conflagrations, may be responsible for partial or total destruc-

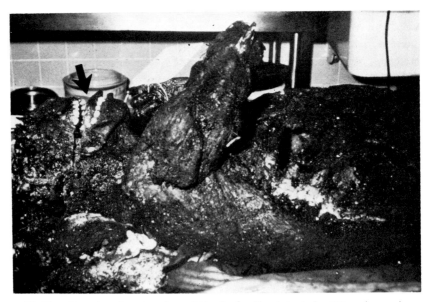

Figure 19. Despite extensive charring of the body, the intact dentition (arrow) persists as an identification medium. AFIP Neg. No. 66-3086-4.

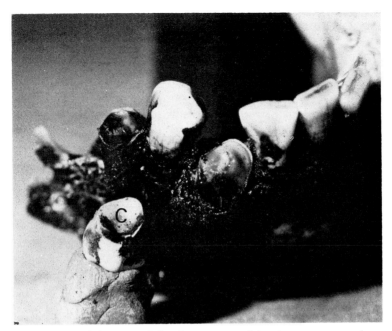

Figure 20. Fire-induced fracture of the dentition resulting in concave regular separation of the exposed crown (C) from the more protected root portion.

tion of dental characteristics. The destructive properties inherent in high-intensity conflagration rest upon two factors: the higher flame temperature and the prolonged duration of exposure. Even in aircraft conflagrations, however, preservation of the dentition is the rule rather than the exception. Details regarding this statement have been provided in Chapter IV.

The soft facial tissues and commonly protruding tongue of conflagration victims serve to protect the teeth from the direct effects of fire and heat (Fig. 19). In fact, a crude impression of tooth outlines may be noted as indentations within the lateral borders of the tongue. The destructive action of conflagration upon the teeth varies from case to case. A rapid exposure to flame may result in a bursting fragmentation of the enamel shell, leaving only the dentin crown structure intact. A more gradual exposure to heat may result in a clean separation at the gum line of the intact crown from the protected cooler root portion which is encased within the jaw structure. Such crown fractures must not be interpreted as being due to blunt trauma (Figs. 20 and 21). Prolonged gradual exposure to heat results in brittleness and an ashen appearance in the dental structures.

As Scott[39] has reported, the heat resistance of the dental metals and plastics varies considerably. Natural teeth can be completely ashed at temperatures of 1000° to 1200° F. The gold alloys (inlays and crowns) commonly

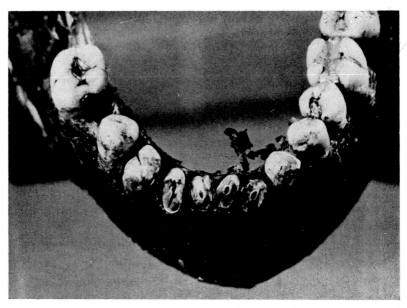

Figure 21. Fire loss of lower anterior crowns. The crown fragments may be located within debris at the fire scene. Such crowns may crumble or be dislodged and lost due to careless handling of the body prior to dental examination.

melt at temperatures of 1600° to 2000° F. Porcelain structures, commonly used in bridgework and as the teeth of some dentures, ordinarily resist temperatures well above 2000° F. The pink acrylic plastic denture bases are consumed at temperatures below those necessary to destroy natural teeth. Amalgam restorations, depending upon their composition, may disappear at low temperatures or may resist destruction at temperatures above 1600° F. Gustafson[40] reports extensively on experimental work regarding dental materials and incineration, and his work should be consulted for further details. The point to be retained in the interpretation of such data is that experimental laboratory situations do not necessarily reflect actual case conditions. The point of fact is that the dentition *in situ* is markedly resistant to the effects of conflagration.

To place this discussion in a practical perspective, it should be stated that household fires rarely reach the level of intensity and duration of conflagration necessary to completely cremate an adult body, dentition included. This is not necessarily true for infant bodies which may be completely destroyed under such conditions. The increased susceptibility of the young body to incineration is due to the decreased body mass and the decreased skeletal calcium salt deposition. It is also difficult to completely cremate an adult body incinerated in a household furnace which often may reach a temperature of 1200° F. In cases where anatomical arrangement of tissues is lost or discernible dental structures cannot be identified, the investigator should not fail to perform radiographic examination of the charred tissue bulk in an effort to disclose teeth, restorations or metallic prostheses. This statement applies not only to the dental aspects of such cases but also to sex, age and race determination from previously unrecognized skeletal structures; the recognition of metallic personal effects; as well as the disclosure of fire-resistant metallic objects (missiles, knife blades) which may indicate that a homicide has occurred.

The dental identification of incinerated bodies has produced many intriguing historical reports. The Parkman-Webster murder in 1849 represents a classic in the annals of forensic odontology.[37, 41] Professor Webster of the Harvard Medical School murdered his friend Doctor Parkman and incinerated the body. Charred jaw bones and dental structures retrieved from Webster's laboratory furnace were identified by Parkman's dentist as being those of the victim. The Goss-Udderzook fraud-murder case occurred in 1872.[42] The Bazar de la Charité and Iroquois Fires represent early examples of mass tragedies wherein identification of remains was accomplished by dental means.[43, 44] Dental fragments served to identify the murdered and burned body in the Carron case; and dental evidence was the means of identification, ten years after death, of the partially burned remains in the Australian Pajama Girl case.[45] The positive identification of Hitler's body was based upon dental comparison.[46] More recently, Sognnaes[47, 48] has discussed the many intriguing aspects of the Hitler, Bormann and Eva Braun identifications.

THE ANTEMORTEM DATA

Earlier in this chapter the antemortem dental data was briefly mentioned. These will now be discussed in detail. The antemortem data of interest are

1. written dental records;
2. dental X rays;
3. casts or models, if available; and
4. recollections of the dentist or acquaintances.

Dental Records of the Attending Dentist

The written dental records maintained by the dentist will usually consist of two elements. The first element is a diagrammatic chart depicting the entire dentition with delineation of the five anatomic surfaces of each tooth (Fig. 22A and B). The tooth diagrams are sufficiently large to enable the dentist to indicate the various restorations, missing teeth and areas of

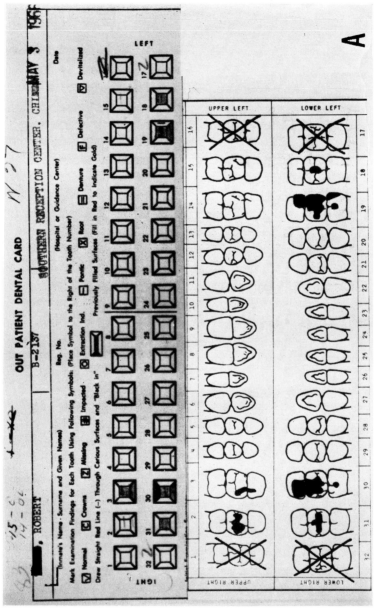

Figure 22A. The upper diagram represents an antemortem outpatient dental record which utilizes a box designation for each tooth and its surfaces. Blackened areas indicate preexisting restorations or decay. The bottom diagram discloses the postmortem charting of the same patient utilizing more anatomic dental figures. Notice the marked superiority of the bottom form enabling much greater characterization of restorations. AFIP Neg. No. 72-11423-1.

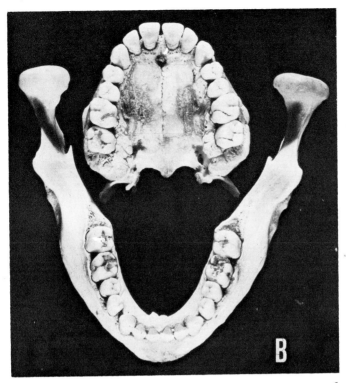

Figure 22B. The dental arches corresponding to the antemortem and postmortem charts of Figure 22A. AFIP Neg. No. 72-12251.

decay. The second element is the area provided for *treatment performed* wherein the dentist's subsequent work will be noted (Fig. 23). Various firms market different dental record forms, but all possess these two basic sections. There are well over forty different tooth numbering systems and symbols; however, the dental chart used by a particular dentist usually contains his numbering system preference in the tooth diagram section of the chart. If questions arise regarding a dentist's numbering method, verification should be made by telephone.

Unfortunately, antemortem dental records are frequently inaccurate, incomplete or confusing. In the ideal situation, the dentist completely charts all preexisting restorations and missing teeth upon the patient's initial visit. This provides a baseline diagram of the dentition. The treatment and alterations thereafter performed by the dentist (and indicated in the treatment performed section) can then be added to the original baseline, and an easily interpreted dental chart is provided for comparison with the postmortem findings. In contrast, one will encounter inadequately maintained charts wherein the original dental status of the patient when first

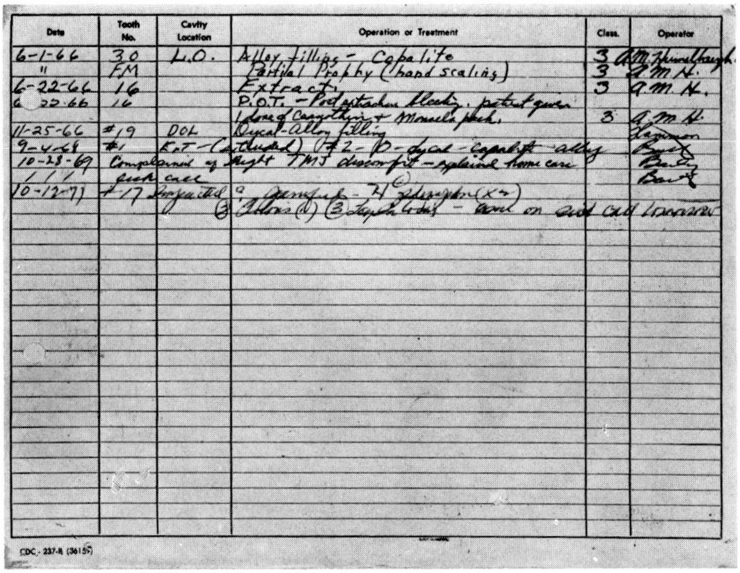

Figure 23. The treatment or work-performed section of the chart for the jaws in Figure 22B. This section indicates procedures done since the patient's initial visit. AFIP Neg. No. 72-11423-2.

seen has not been recorded and only subsequent treatment has been noted. In such an instance, unless all the work in the patient's mouth has been performed by the dentist submitting the records, many valuable points (in the form of preexisting restorations) necessary for comparison are eliminated, and the total comparison may be invalid or lack specificity. Hopefully, in such cases initial or subsequent dental X rays may salvage the situation. Another common situation is that the dentist may indicate only his own work in the tooth diagram section. The person performing dental identification must be aware of the various inconsistencies in the manner of charting and must interpret these in relation to the particular case at hand.[36]

It is important to obtain the inclusive dates of treatment and of the dating of dental X rays since this may be of importance in the subsequent comparison. Usually this information will be provided in the treatment performed area of the chart.

The identification expert should keep in mind that many city, state or federal institutions maintain dental care facilities for their subjects, including penal institutions, mental hospitals and Veterans Administration (VA) treatment centers. A search of such facilities in a putative identity with such a background may be quite fruitful. In addition, complete dentures constructed by these facilities may contain an embedded name or identifying number. For putative identities with a history of service in the U.S. military, the possibility of filed dental records on the deceased should be checked with the Military Personnel Records Center in St. Louis, Missouri.

It should be kept in mind that many persons utilize the services of several dentists or dental specialists during their lifetime. If the examiner locates a dentist in reference to a putative identity, this dentist should also be questioned regarding the knowledge of any other dentists who may have provided care to the deceased. In a similar context, the family may know only of a physician who provided care to the deceased. On occasion, the physician may have the patient's dentist on record.

Dental X rays

Dental X rays are a valuable asset for comparison studies. They are of utmost necessity in the presence of an inadequate antemortem dental chart. X rays not only supplement or correct the written record, but they delineate the specific morphology of restorations as well as provide insight into many facets of comparison not visible on oral examination. Such points of comparison include intertooth relationships, root angulation, tooth and pulp canal outlines, jawbone trabecular pattern, periapical (about the root apex) pathology, root canal therapy (endodontia) (Figs. 8 and 9) and retained root tips which may have remained following previous loss of teeth. In addition, interproximal bone loss due to periodontal (gum) disease and rarely encountered jawbone pathologic processes also may serve as entities for comparison. The X-ray comparison, of course, is between the antemortem X rays and dental X rays performed as part of the postmortem examination (see Chap. VI). Such a comparison may enable positive identification to be made upon one or several teeth which otherwise reveal only nonspecific restorations upon examination by the naked eye.

The proper viewing and mounting of dental X rays may present some difficulty to those unfamiliar with such techniques. A commonly used means of viewing X rays will be presented here. Dental X rays are viewed from the lingual aspect, that is, as though one were inside the mouth looking out. Intraoral X rays are easily recognized as upper or lower, right or left, by observing the following:

1. The film should be viewed with the shiny side toward the examiner. Many films will have an embossed dot in one corner; the depressed surface of this dot should be facing the viewer. These features indicate the lingual aspect of the teeth observed. The observer will therefore be looking at the X rays as though he were inside the mouth looking out.

2. The anatomy of the respective teeth indicate upper or lower dentition. The upper anterior teeth have the broad central and narrow lateral incisors. The lower anteriors reveal the four incisors of about the same width. The upper posterior teeth may disclose the maxillary sinus superimposed about the root apices. The upper molars usually possess three roots compared to the bi-rooted lower molars. The occlusal line of the upper posterior teeth forms a gentle upward arching line (the curve of Spee).

3. The laterality, right or left, is determined by the distal aspect of the film. If the distal lies on the right, the view is of the right side. If the distal is to the left, the view is of the left side.

It will be recalled that the dental metals show up as radiopacities. The nonmetal silicate and acrylic restorations, used on anterior teeth, are radiolucent and may appear as dental decay. Root canal fillings (either metallic or cones) are radiopaque. Periapical abscesses are radiolucent provided the lateral bony plates of the respective jaw have been thinned or perforated.

Also one should recall that the chronologic age of the postmortem remains (in persons less than 22-24 years of age) can more accurately be determined by the X ray than by mere naked-eye observation of the erupted teeth. The reason for this is that the X ray portrays the precise stage of root calcification (see Chaps. II and VIII).

In the absence of a known attending dentist or of antemortem dental records, the examiner should not fail to consider the possibility of previous skull X rays that may have been performed on the putative deceased. Such X rays are usually retained in a hospital X-ray department film library. Skull X rays, although not as definitive as dental X rays, may still provide the information necessary for identification purposes.

Dental Casts or Models

Dental casts or models are exact replicas of a patient's dentition and are invaluable for comparison with the postmortem remains. Such stone casts, prepared from impressions of the teeth, may have been constructed for purposes of the manufacture of prosthetic devices, for crown restorations or for orthodontic (braces) therapy. Unfortunately, such casts are not usually retained by the dentist or dental laboratory once they have served their purpose. On occasion the patient may have been given the model as a souvenir or keepsake, and the family should be questioned regarding this possibility if necessary. Such casts are also constructed for full denture procedures, and even the edentulous (toothless) cast can be matched with the remains or with a postmortem cast regarding specific features such as the alveolar ridge contour and dimensions as well as the palatal rugae configuration (Figs. 24 and 25).

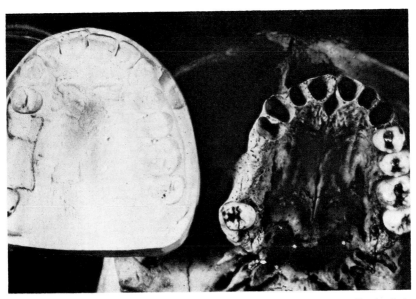

Figure 24. A stone cast (left) and the corresponding skeletonized maxilla (right). Note the postmortem loss of anterior teeth from the skeleton. The right posterior segment of the cast identically matches the dimensions of the skeleton regarding this area of old tooth loss.

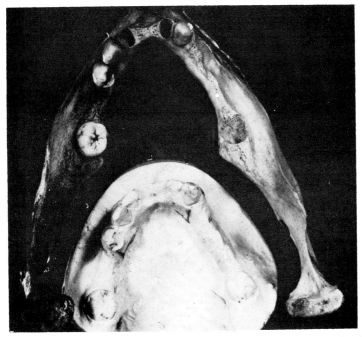

Figure 25. The mandible and corresponding cast of the Figure 24 case also disclose an exact comparison regarding arch configuration and tooth loss.

Recollection of the Dentition

On occasion, the dentist's memory may be sufficient to provide quite specific antemortem data. The author recalls contacting the dentist of an unidentified air crash victim who had discarded the records in question eight years earlier. Nevertheless, the dentist exactly described several areas of bridgework which matched in every detail the postmortem findings. The dentist related that he would never forget the work since it represented his first case of extensive bridgework following entry into private practice.

On rare occasions the dentist may have photographs of the dentition available.

Although far from providing a scientific account of the dental arches, family members or friends may recollect particularly striking abnormalities of the dentition of the decedent. Such information may be of value in assisting identification in conjunction with other methods or in establishing identification by the teeth if the particular alteration is specific (Figs. 26A and B).

Occasionally, the postmortem dental examiner will encounter an attending dentist who refuses to cooperate in the comparison. Such withholding of information may result from several aroused anxieties. The attending dentist may possess fears of becoming involved in a bizarre legal hassle, which, of course, is merely a precipitate of his own ignorance regarding the role of dentistry and identification. The author has recently seen a case where resistance was encountered due to suspected previous insurance payments made to the attending dentist for work noted in the chart which, in fact, was never performed on the patient. Although such instances are rare, one should keep in mind that even though the dental records are the rightful legal property of the dentist, such records may be subpoenaed by the investigating authorities. Almost in every instance, however, the decedent's dentist is pleased to be of any assistance and will strive in any way to contribute.

In the retrieval of antemortem records, it is important to obtain the most recent records regarding the dental care afforded the patient. This applies to cases where the decedent has received care from several dentists. If only an earlier record is available, irresolvable incompatibilities and inconsistencies may plague the comparison due to the alterations induced by the subsequently performed dental work.

In summation, from the standpoint of antemortem information, effectual dental identification necessitates

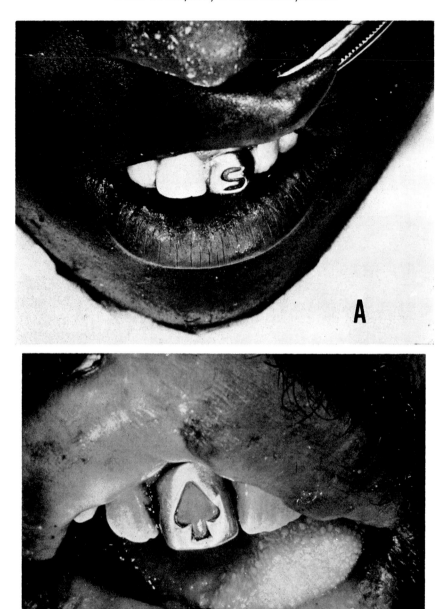

Figure 26. Characterized anterior crowns of two subjects readily recalled by acquaintances. Such dental findings substantiate less reliable identification data (as personal effects) and enable positive scientific identification.

1. a putative (suspected) identity of the unknown body or bodies in question and
2. the availability of recent and accurate antemortem data for comparison.

Chapter VI

PROCEDURAL ASPECTS OF THE POSTMORTEM DENTAL EXAMINATION

GENERAL CONSIDERATIONS

UNDER IDEAL CIRCUMSTANCES, the postmortem dental examination should begin at the site where the body is found. This statement is made because police and fire department officials are not expected to recognize dental remains as they commonly exist under conditions surrounding the decomposed, charred or traumatically mutilated body. Furthermore, in the author's experience, such individuals are often not cognizant of the role that a single dislodged tooth, jaw fragment or dental appliance may play in any eventual identification. In contrast to the usual identification format as exists in this country, Norway, by law, has an established identification committee consisting of a law enforcement officer, physician and dentist who jointly participate in the identification procedures applied to any disaster situation which results in fatalities.[49]

In the United States, common practice indicates that the dentist or pathologist is not involved with case identification until the body is located in a mortuary facility. On occasion, such a practice will result in loss of dental structures at the scene amidst debris and vegetation or in loss of dental items during body transport. The presence of a dentist at the scene is especially desired in the mass disaster situation. The ideal is to have the dentist survey the body at the scene, superficially view the oral structures at the time if feasible and search the immediate vicinity for any obviously lost dental elements.

In circumstances involving several bodies, any such recovered items should be marked as to site location and placed in a plastic bag labeled according to an adjacent body number or a grid location. The actual charting of a mass disaster or homicide scene does not fall within the responsibility of the dentist; so he need not be concerned with such details. The on-scene dental consultant must realize that his activities are under the direction of the governing coroner, pathologist or law enforcement official; and he must appreciate the fact that although his goal may represent a significant aspect of the investigation, it still occupies but a small segment of the total situation and maze of problems that are developing amid the surroundings. The dentist will work most intimately with the medical personnel assisting or regulating the investigation.

Once the body or bodies have been removed to a morgue facility, the dentist will find himself in a more comfortable familiar environment and will by then be assigned to the specific role of assisting in the identification procedure.

Depending upon the circumstances and the manpower available, the dentist may be expected to assist other parties in the cataloging of identifying items (i.e. the patient's clothing, jewelry and personal effects) in addition to his assigned task of dental identification. Such assistance by the dentist is usually greatly appreciated at such times.

The dental charting should include all of the features mentioned in the following chapter (see Chap. VII). Most routine identifications are accomplished on the basis of the pattern of missing teeth and restorations, prostheses and decay. It should be stressed that such identifications can be competently handled by the forensic pathologist or physician provided he has devoted some time and energy to the understanding of basic principles of dentistry, dental materials and dental nomenclature. The physician or pathologist can easily learn to master the techniques of comparison pertinent to the process of dental identification. As discussed in Chapter I, it is advisable that the larger medical examiner systems in this country establish a working relationship with a dentist or group of dentists interested in assisting with the more complex problems inherent to forensic dentistry. Such instances include cases where confusing data complicate the comparison procedure. A mass disaster situation almost surely demands a team approach to the identification problem as elucidated and stressed in Chapter IV. In any emergency crisis, there is no better safeguard to effectiveness than preparedness. This certainly applies to the topic of mass disasters.

It should be reemphasized at this point that the field of dental identification must be retained in its proper position regarding the total identification format (see Chap. III). It is impractical to immediately effect dental identification procedures on every unknown body that enters the medical examiner's or coroner's office unless it is obvious from the outset that other acceptable methods of identification will be useless. Generally speaking, little can be accomplished from the dental examination until a putative identity is forwarded; obviously, the passage of time does not alter the dental structures. It is best to sit back, gather general data regarding the circumstances of death and identity, record the personal effects and autopsy data and correlate all such information with investigating police officials. In the meantime, the fingerprint method of identification can be initiated if feasible. At a later stage, if necessary, the dental examination can be performed either to establish positive identity or to substantially corroborate or dispute an established or putative identification. Of course, a set identification format cannot be predicated for each and every case; however, the fact remains that the pursuit of antemortem dental records without a greatly narrowed putative population segment is an extensive chore resulting in needless expenditure of time and effort.

If, in the last analysis, identification of the body remains unknown, the dental structures should always be removed *en bloc* and retained in formalin containers with the corresponding autopsy number attached. Such an unidentified body will eventually be removed, whether it be for cremation, Anatomy Board disposition or *Potters Field* burial. The retention of dental structures offers the possibility of positive identification months or years later should subsequent information and dental records regarding the identity evolve. *En bloc* jaw resection is easier, less expensive, less time-consuming and more accurate than the construction of stone models from dental impressions.

THE EXAMINATION

A handy dental identification kit should be available for use in any medical examiner facility and/or by any dentist with an interest in the field of dental identification. Such kits are inexpensive, can be purchased in any dental supply house and can be tailored to the personal needs of the particular dentist. Such a kit is depicted in Figure 27. The reader should keep in mind that in addition to the items available in the kit, a portable battery-operated headlamp, gauze sponges for cleansing the teeth, heavy-duty autopsy gloves and dental charts must be taken to the on-scene investigations. Photographic and tape-recording equipment are optional accessories.

The fact that bodies requiring dental identification are frequently disfigured due to trauma or decomposition obviates the possibility of funeral viewing by relatives and allows the examiner to dissect and remove the facial and jaw structures at will to permit a proper effectual examination.

Depending upon the individual case, the examiner may elect to incise only the cheek structures to gain proper intraoral access or may decide to remove the jaw structures *en bloc*. The latter procedure utilizes an electrical autopsy saw for removal of the bony structures and enables proper cleansing of the teeth and accurate registration of the postmortem data. It also provides excellent exposure for any desired photographic purposes. Removal of the jaws is accomplished by a horizontal saw cut through the maxilla parallel to the occlusal plane of the teeth. For the mandible, bilateral horizontal saw cuts through the rami will allow jaw removal fol-

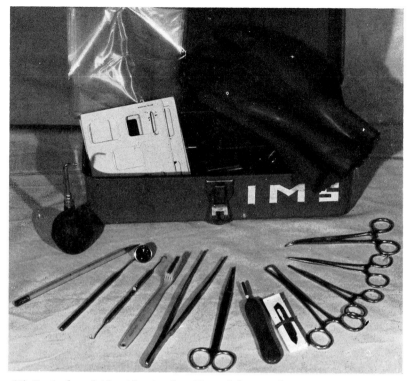

Figure 27. Basic dental identification kit. From left to right: air syringe, pencil, mirror, explorer, toothbrush, tissue forceps, scissors, scalpel handle and blades, tongue clamp and hemostats (3). Autopsy gloves, polyethylene bags and dental X ray film holder are seen in the case. For examinations performed outside of the autopsy room, be sure that gauze sponges (for tooth cleansing), a source of illumination (flashlight or headlamp) and the dental examination form are included.

lowing scalpel release of the floor of the soft mouth tissues. An autopsy hammer and chisel set, available in any mortuary facility, may be necessary for bone separation. If one elects to preserve the jaws for a museum or for teaching or photographic purposes, a scalpel should be used to trim off as much soft tissue as possible and the jaw structures should be placed in a 5% sodium hypochlorite solution (bleach) for several hours. The end result of the removal and cleansing of the jaws as described is seen in Figures 12 and 13 of Chapter II.

In mass disaster situations, the removal of the jaws and their placement in transparent labeled plastic bags provides for easy, subsequent review of the findings for comparison purposes. Once the jaws are removed, the examiner may elect to retire to more comfortable quarters for the dental charting procedure. The jaws can later be reunited with the proper body for burial purposes. For the identification of cases involving but a single body, intraoral examination is usually sufficient.

In cases involving recently deceased bodies where facial features are preserved and rigor mortis prevents adequate opening of the mouth, it is inadvisable to mutilate the head for purposes of oral examination. In these instances one should either incise the masticatory muscles from within the oral cavity or *break* the rigor by leverage employing a rongeur inserted into the retromolar spaces bilaterally. In the latter procedure care must be exercised so as not to fracture or loosen the dentition. A mouth prop may then be inserted to maintain the mouth in an open position. An alternative is to wait until rigor mortis has disappeared (usually 20-30 hours postmortem), at which time the jaws are relaxed.

Any dislodged teeth should be secured into the appropriate mouth position by use of an adhesive cement. This is best accomplished at the examination facility (rather than at the scene of death) where better lighting conditions prevail to insure that each tooth is placed in the proper socket. A collection of such teeth at the scene should include tooth placement in suitable containers or bags for transferral to the examination site. This especially applies to a multiple body situation where isolated dental remnants should be labeled as to an adjacent body or designated via a grid location in reference to the map of the total scene. It is important that the dentist assume the responsibility of tooth placement as it is rather easy to place a dislodged tooth into the wrong alveolar socket. The dentist's experience, as compared to that of nondental personnel, lessens this possibility.

Under ideal conditions, the dental examination should be performed by two persons, one actually performing the examination and one recording the data. Both individuals should be thoroughly familiar with dental terminology. It is important that the recorder view the actual teeth to accurately demarcate the morphological pattern of the restorations or areas of decay. The examiner should also review the completed chart. Two persons, functioning as a team, provide more accurate and cleaner records and also work faster. The time factor is especially important in mass disaster situations where anxious relatives and news media are pressing for identification. If a pre-established dental team is not available, local dental societies or dental schools are usually more than willing to assist at times of mass disaster. Advanced dental school students serve as excellent recorders.

The postmortem dental chart need not be complex and should include adequate space for depiction of restoration morphology. The chart currently employed by the Office of the Chief Medical Examiner, State of Maryland, is a modification of the Department of Defense Form 891 (Fig. 28) and adequately meets the needs for purposes of dental identification. A more complex and most thorough dental examination chart has been devised by Curtis Mertz, the consultant forensic odontologist for the Ohio Highway Patrol in Ashtabula, Ohio.

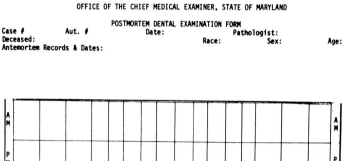

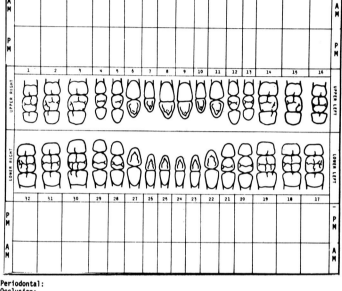

Figure 28. Postmortem dental examination form. AM-antemortem data; PM-postmortem charting.

In the performance of the postmortem examination notation, a mark should be designated for each of the thirty-two teeth on the chart. Even if a tooth is unremarkable (normal), the tooth should be so designated. It is also important to indicate which jaw segments were not recovered or whether missing teeth are the result of postmortem or antemortem loss. Such notations are vital to the efficient screening of the postmortem data when compared with antemortem records. There should be an area of the chart reserved for the final conclusions of the dentist. This area should include any remarks by the dentist which explain any inconsistencies and may enable positive identification from otherwise superficially unmatching features. One must remember that the identification expert may be called upon several months later to testify regarding his findings, at which time specific details concerning these matters may not be readily apparent. As examples, such explanations should include mention of *drifting molars* (see Chap. VII), X-ray findings which correct a poor chart or records, etc.

It is imperative that the name and address of the antemortem dentist who supplied the records be retained as part of the official record. The dates of treatment and X rays should also be recorded. In addition, if the circumstances of the case initially indicate that subsequent court testimony regarding the identification may be forthcoming (as in the homicide victim), the dentist may wish to copy the originally submitted records and X rays for retention in the case folder. X-ray duplication is accomplished by use of a photographic printing frame and Kodak Radiograph Duplicating Film®. Specific details can be obtained from a photographic supply dealer.

Photographs of the examined postmortem dentition are not essential but serve to substantiate the postmortem record and provide excellent lecture material for teaching purposes. This is most easily accomplished in resected jaw specimens; however, mirrors can be employed for adequate photographs of the jaws *in situ*. A good 35mm camera with color transparency film and a light source is all that is required. A macrolens (close-up lens) is advisable. Most hospital autopsy rooms or medical examiner facilities have photographic equipment readily available as part of their standard operation.

MULTIPLE BODY IDENTIFICATION

In multiple body identification, the format should initially segregate the remains into subcategories as to sex and age where possible. This task involves collaboration between the pathologist, dentist and other persons (usually police personnel) involved in the identification procedure. Such categorization immediately narrows the population segment applicable to any particular body. Such segregation, of course, is based upon visual recognition of body parts or physical features, recovered personal effects and clothing and the results of the complete postmortem examination. It must be kept in mind that despite a totally charred or mutilated body exterior, the internal organs are generally preserved to enable an assessment to be made regarding sex, approximate age of the deceased, missing organs and even homicidal injuries if applicable. Such data should eventually be amalgamated into elimination charts as devised by Delaney in the Noronic disaster.[35] Keep in mind that the dental identification may prove to be the conclusive or only mode of identification of a victim(s), depending, of course, upon the total circumstances. If dental identification methods are instituted, the preliminary breakdown of bodies into sex and age followed by basic dental categories based upon the presence of full or partial dentures, of bridgework and of gold restorations enables the comparison format to concentrate upon already established subpopulations. The subsequent retrieval of antemortem data will then enable rapid identification of such subpopulations. The most difficult identifications are those based upon comparisons of the patterns of the common amalgam restorations and missing teeth. They represent the bulk of cases in a multiple body situation and are also the most time-consuming comparisons.

The dentist may prefer to remove the jaws from the body as described earlier, clean the specimens, label bags with the appropriate body number and subsequently retire to another area to perform his examination. Postmortem dental radiographs can also be effected upon such removed jaw specimens and eliminate the difficulty of moving entire bodies about for purposes of radiologic examination. The Canadian group utilized 35mm color transparencies in their comparison procedures.[21]

The ideal cases for comparison are those wherein the dental arches are recovered intact in their entirety and where accurate, up-to-date antemortem records are available. Given time, such cases become rather straightforward identifications. The problem cases arise when only portions of the dentition remain and poor antemortem records, or none at all, can be located. In the comparison procedure, the problem cases should be left for last, a format which will allow the elimination of the easier comparisons leaving a small number of unmatched antemortem records for consideration.

In the mass disaster situation, if it is apparent from the outset that dental identification procedures are necessary or desirable, immediate efforts should commence, based upon the list of putative identities (such as in an air crash), to locate the antemortem dental records and to have them transferred to the site where the examination is being performed. A dentist should be involved in any telephone contact with the antemortem dentist, since police or other nondental personnel are unfamiliar with dental terminology or charting procedures. Dentist-to-dentist communication will provide immediate transferral of data; and subsequent copies of antemortem charts or X rays can be relayed, if necessary, by mail or police messenger.

The reader should keep in mind the fact that mass disasters involving many children of the same approximate age[12, 25, 26] or large numbers of patients possessing complete dentures[18, 23] may present difficulties due to the fact that gross differential features of these dentitions may be minimal.

POSTMORTEM DENTAL RADIOGRAPHS

The postmortem dental radiograph is used to enhance points of comparison and to reveal certain dental findings which are not visible upon naked-eye, oral examination. The latter findings commonly include the performance of endodontic treatment, retained root tips as the result of previous loss of teeth and the presence of impacted teeth. The use of the X ray is mandatory for the estimation of chronologic age based upon the degree of root calcification and/or the status of unerupted teeth (see Chap. VIII). In addition, the postmortem X ray of the dental restoration enables a distinct comparison to be made regarding the morphology of the filling material as compared on the antemortem and postmortem X ray films (see Fig. 52). The comparison of antemortem and postmortem X rays also enables innumerable concordant points to be established regarding root curvature angulation, root canal and pulp chamber outlines, and bone patterns, provided specific characteristics are noted. The postmortem dental X ray often enables one to settle any *drifting molar* inconsistency (see Chap. VII) because the mesial drift of the second or third molar into the position of a lost first or second molar, respectively, will be noted by the mesial lean or drift of the involved tooth (see Fig. 32).

The procedure of taking postmortem dental X rays is not difficult and requires little practice to achieve success provided one standardizes his equipment regarding exposure time and Kvp settings. The settings will vary depending upon the machine and film utilized. Depending upon the individual machine, it may be possible to use the standard autopsy room medical X-ray unit for dental radiographs. Experimentation or consultation with a radiologist or radiology technician may be necessary. It is preferable to purchase a second-hand inexpensive dental X-ray unit which is far more flexible and more easily manipulated than the large medical X-ray unit. Intraoral dental radiographic film and plastic or cardboard film mounts can be purchased at any dental supply house. Dental radiographs can also be developed in any standard X-ray darkroom. The procedure of mounting the fixed X rays has already been described (see Chap. V).

In taking the intraoral X ray, the film is placed on the lingual or palatal side of the teeth and can be maintained in position using plastic dental X-ray film holders or self-constructed small wooden film holders. In skeletal remains, the film can be retained in position using masking tape or plasticine. Because the angulation of the X ray in relation to the tooth and film will determine the degree of distortion of the true image, for the comparison of specific features (such as restoration morphology or bone pattern), it is best to approximate the angulation employed by the dentist in taking the antemortem radiograph. This can best be accomplished by directing the path of the X ray so that it is perpendicular to a plane bisecting the angle formed by the vertical axis of the tooth and the vertical axis of the X ray film. This sounds more complicated than it actually is, and experimentation is the best means of establishing perfection. In fact, reasonably intelligent autopsy room dieners can easily be taught the technique of postmortem dental radiography.

Chapter VII

THE POSTMORTEM DENTAL DATA

THE COMMON POSTMORTEM POINTS OF COMPARISON

IT SHOULD BE CLEAR by this time that any deviation from the normal anatomic configuration of the oral structures or any alteration of the virginal status of the endowed dentition represents potential grist for the mill of the person performing dental identification. The common parameters which bear features of specificity and which should be observed are

1. the number of teeth,
2. restorations and prostheses,
3. decay (dental caries),
4. malposition and malrotation,
5. peculiar shapes of teeth,
6. root canal therapy (endodontia),
7. bone patterns,
8. complete dentures,
9. relationship of the bite,
10. oral pathology,
11. occupational changes and socioeconomic pattern of the dentition and
12. sex and race determination.

The reader should realize that most dental identifications are established upon the first three parameters, that is, the location of missing teeth and the location and surface involvement of restorations, bridgework and caries. Each of the above parameters will be discussed in turn.

The Number of Teeth

Absence of Teeth

Missing teeth may be a result of therapeutic extraction, natural tooth loss, traumatic tooth loss or congenital absence. On occasion, the distinction between recent antemortem and postmortem tooth loss is of major significance.

THERAPEUTIC EXTRACTION: This term refers to teeth removed by the dentist for reasons of improving the oral health of the patient. Common indications for extraction include:

1. abscessed teeth,

2. symptomatic or asymptomatic nonrestorable teeth due to caries activity,

3. periodontal (gum) conditions which result in tooth-supportive bone loss and excessive tooth mobility (common in the middle-aged and the elderly),

4. the removal of healthy teeth to alleviate or prevent an existing or expected crowding of the dental arch (most commonly practiced in the under-15 age group). Such extractions usually involve the primary molars and/or the permanent premolars.

NATURAL TOOTH LOSS: The reference here is to tooth loss as a result of numbers 1, 2 or 3 above in the absence of dental treatment. Such loss is common in persons of lower socioeconomic status and often is noted in mouths showing other features of dental neglect such as untreated caries or periodontal disease (pyorrhea). Not infrequently the entire crown portion of a tooth (usually molars or premolars) will be broken away due to the combined effects of caries and masticatory forces exerted upon the weakened crown structure. In such instances, only protruding root structures may be evident (Fig. 29). It is not possible to differentiate therapeu-

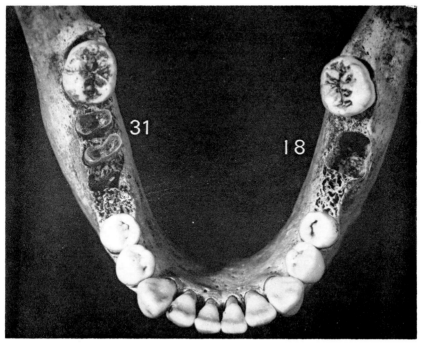

Figure 29. Mandible showing only root tips for tooth 31. Also note postmortem and remote tooth loss for areas 18 and 19, respectively. Such a jaw indicates poor dental care and correlates with low socioeconomic status.

tic versus natural tooth loss in cases where the tooth has been completely removed and healing of the tooth socket has ensued.

TRAUMATIC TOOTH LOSS: This term, of course, applies to the effects of blunt-force injury as a result of a fall or blow. It also applies almost exclusively to the anterior teeth. In cases of healed dental injury there is usually no indication of the fact that the tooth loss was trauma-induced. In instances of more extensive old facial trauma, of course, gross jawbone and soft-tissue deformity and scars may indicate such an event.

CONGENITAL ABSENCE OF TEETH: The congenital absence of teeth results from the lack of tooth bud formation (see Chap. III). The teeth usually involved are the third molars, the second premolars and the maxillary lateral incisors.

IMPACTED MOLARS AND TOOTH DRIFT: Upon consideration of absent teeth, two phenomena require elucidation since they may present confusing inconsistencies in the comparison. The first of these phenomena is the entity of *impacted teeth*. Impacted teeth are not visible upon naked-eye oral examination; but in fact, these teeth are present although trapped and submerged within the jawbone or covered by the gingival tissue. Most commonly, this process involves the third molars. The third molars, the last teeth to erupt into the mouth, frequently are victimized by the evolutionary shortening of the jaw structure so that there is inadequate space for their vertical eruption into the dental arch. The eruption of these teeth is thereby prevented, and they may remain forever embedded within the jawbone. The appreciation and recognition of this phenomenon is of importance when an approximate age estimation is being established on the basis of erupted teeth only. The unrecognized existence of impacted third molars (commonly a bilateral process) may lead to the false conclusion that the subject is less than seventeen to twenty-one years of age when, in fact, the subject may be considerably older. In a case presenting with grossly absent third molars, X rays of the third-molar regions are necessary to evaluate the actual presence (the teeth may have been previously extracted) and calcification status of these teeth. Only in this manner can the dental age be estimated. The apices of the third molars fully calcify and fuse at about twenty to twenty-two years of age (see Chap. VIII). The following case serves to illustrate the determination of dental age based upon third-molar root formation:

> An unknown skeleton was found in an abandoned warehouse. The scene investigation (belt around neck suspended from a rafter) suggested that the manner of death was suicide. A general anthropologic survey of the skeleton indicated that the bones in question were from a Negro female in her late teens. The dentition was intact and served to further estimate the age as well as to effect specific identification.

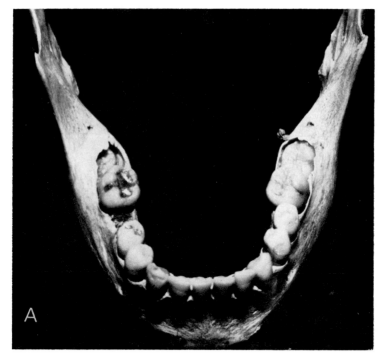

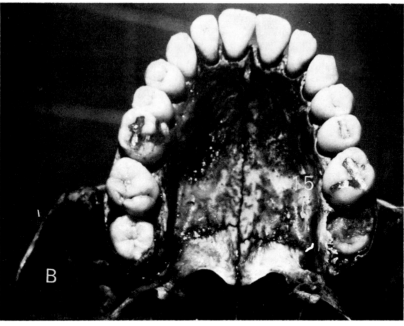

Figure 30. A. Note unerupted third molars suggestive of a person less than seventeen years of age. The left side shows distal drifting of the premolars as they close the gap following loss of the first molar several years earlier. B. The maxilla also reveals unerupted third molars. Note complete mesial drift of the left second molar (15) to obliterate space of the lost first molar in the distant past. The dentist antemortem may erroneously regard such a tooth as the first molar (14) when it is, in fact, the second molar (15).

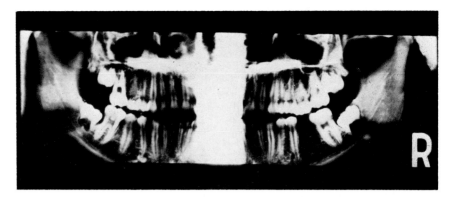

Figure 31. A postmortem panoramic X ray (teeth 1 and 32 on the right) shows incomplete root formation of all third molars. Note the mesial drift of the lower left second molar (18) completely closing the gap of the missing first molar.

The third molars were still partially encased in the respective jaw bones in an unerupted state (Fig. 30A and B). Roentgenographic examination of the third molars indicated root formation comparable to that expected for a person of approximately 15½ years of age plus/minus one year (Figs. 31 and 32). Further examination of the teeth revealed that the nature and neatness of the restorations were indicative of their placement by a most conscientious dentist, possibly in a public school clinic. A tentative identification was subsequently established by correlating the estimated age, sex, race, interval since death and nature of the clothing with a listing of the Missing Persons Bureau. This tentative identification was verified by comparison with the antemortem dental records located at the dental clinic where the girl had attended school. Had the Missing Persons Bureau not led to the putative identity in this case, we had proposed to investigate the nearby neighborhoods for school clinics on the assumption that the girl probably had lived in the area where the body was discovered. Once the case was completed the relative locations of the home, the warehouse and the school clinic were noted to be within a six-block radius of each other. The adolescent had passed her sixteenth birthday on the day prior to her disappearance and was extremely dejected at not receiving any presents as well as recently being rejected by a boyfriend.

A second phenomenon which may present as an inconsistency in the dental comparison is the concept of *drifting molars*. This term refers to the fact that upon the loss of a molar tooth, a subsequently erupting or erupted molar may drift forward (mesially) to occupy the space previously occupied by the removed tooth. The mesial shifting of this molar is due to the fact that teeth in normal alignment serve to stabilize the position of a particular tooth relative to each of its neighbors. The situation can be compared to the mutual support of closely spaced slats of a picket fence. If an adjacent neighboring tooth is lost, this support function fails and the remaining tooth or teeth adjacent to the gap will then follow the path of least resistance under the seige of masticatory forces and tip or drift toward the open space.

The most common situation is one wherein the first permanent molar (6-year molar) is lost early in life with the subsequent partial or total drift of the second molar (12-year molar) into the space previously occupied by the first molar (Fig. 30A and B). Upon naked-eye examination, the antemortem dentist may have thereby erroneously recorded the second molar as the first molar, and any subsequent caries or restorations noted regarding the tooth will be improperly assigned to the first molar. The postmortem examiner, with a better view of the dentition and with the aid of a postmortem radiograph (which will usually reveal a mesial tipping or

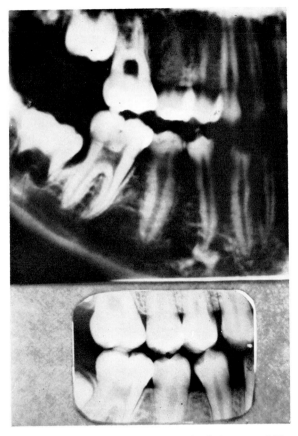

Figure 32. The upper X ray is an enlargement of the left jaws of Figure 31. Note the lack of root formation of the lower third molar in comparison to the fully formed second molar. The dental age was estimated at 15.5 years. The lower X ray was taken shortly before death. Note the favorable comparison of the backward (distal) angulation of the lower first premolar (21) on both X rays.

drift of the second molar), will correctly recognize the tooth as being the second molar (and not the first molar as recorded by the antemortem dentist); and thus, an apparent mismatch will be recognized as an inconsistency and not as an incompatibility (Figs. 31 and 32). The problem of drifting molars is not infrequent and most commonly involves the mesial drift of the second molar into the first-molar position. Less commonly, the third molar may drift into the slot of a previously lost second molar. The postmortem examiner should be especially cognizant of the drifting concept in cases where all of the points of comparison are concordant except for a first molar/second molar or second molar/third molar discrepancy.

ANTEMORTEM VS. POSTMORTEM TOOTH LOSS: The postmortem loss of teeth is by no means infrequent and results from deterioration of the soft-tissue periodontal ligaments responsible for securing the tooth within the alveolus (socket). The tooth-socket relationship is, in actuality, a joint stabilized by fibrous tissue (the periodontal membrane). The finding is noted in decomposed bodies, especially those submerged in water, and almost always to some degree in skeletal remains. Postmortem loss usually involves anterior teeth with inverted conical roots so that such teeth easily fall out or become dislodged by movement. The double- and triple-rooted teeth, such as the molars and upper premolars, due to their root curvature, are less commonly displaced postmortem.

In nondecomposed remains, the exposed socket of a tooth lost postmortem will be free of blood clots and will reveal no evidence of vital hemorrhage regarding adjacent gingival trauma or lip contusion as might be expected in cases of perimortem trauma. In addition, any tongue injury also is free of vital reaction.

An associated jaw fracture (mandible or premaxilla) may be evident with or without the loss of teeth in instances of trauma occurring antemortem, perimortem or postmortem. The timing of these latter injuries may be dated by the usual gross and microscopic criteria applied to dating of injuries. One should keep in mind that a lateral blow to the mandible (such as a swinging fist) may fracture not only the body of the mandible on the side of the blow (usually in the premolar area) but also the contralateral condyle neck as a result of force transmitted to the latter structure by the upward displacement or *plunger effect* of the strongly ligamentous supported temporomandibular joint. Violent midline mandibular impact in the mental region (as seen in auto accidents) may drive both condyles into their respective glenoid fossae resulting in transverse bilateral middle fossa skull fractures with or without associated mandibular fractures.

In the recently deceased, the observation of a clot within the socket implies recent antemortem tooth loss, traumatic or otherwise. Histologic sections are required for age estimation of the wound (described below). In circumstances of possible homicide, such an examination may be pertinent to the reconstruction of events surrounding the death. In an unidentified body, such a finding may indicate recent dental care.

Postmortem tooth loss in skeletal remains presents as a clean, smooth socket wall with a feathered, sharp alveolar rim. In contrast, recent or old antemortem tooth loss as noted in the skeleton results in varying degrees of bone remodeling from rounding of the rim in early repair to a complete fill-in of the socket with secondary bone formation. Such bony repair begins at the base and periphery of the socket so that the crest of the bone is remodeled and calcified last (Fig. 33). Within three to five months following tooth loss, new bone formation fills the socket; however, the alveolar outline may still be visible on X-ray examination. Within six months to one year following tooth loss, complete bony obliteration of the alveolus is noted; however, slight depression of the alveolar ridge outline will persist (Figs. 34 and 35). On occasion, the stage of healing of an extraction site may be vital to an identification case wherein it is known that recent antemortem tooth loss occurred. The basic histologic reparative fea-

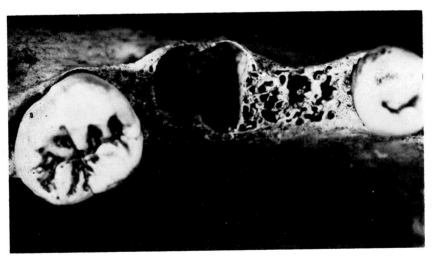

Figure 33. Lower left jaw showing postmortem tooth loss characterized by a socket with a sharp rim or edge. The adjacent mesial space shows almost complete remodeling of what was once a socket for the first molar. The latter tooth had been lost antemortem in the remote past. This figure is an enlargement of Figure 29. AFIP Neg. No. 73-1981-2.

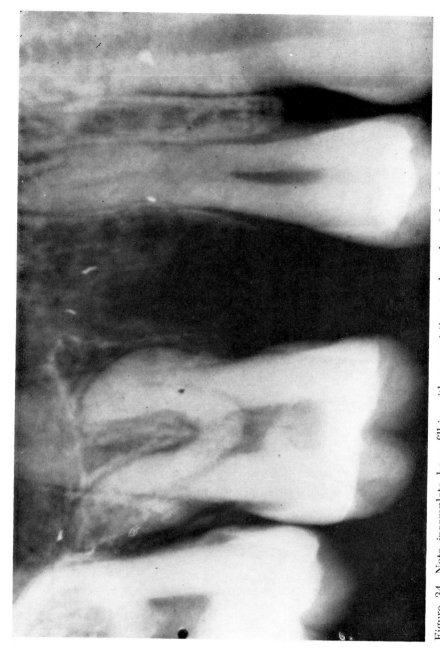

Figure 34. Note incomplete bone fill-in with a persisting tooth socket (alveolus) outline 2.5 months after extraction.

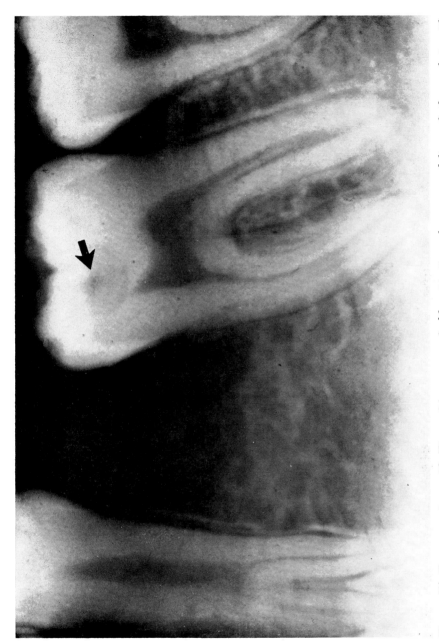

Figure 35. For comparison with Figure 34, an area of old extraction shows remodeling of the socket with complete bone fill-in and loss of alveolar outline. Also note mesial drift and tipping of the molar. The molar also contains decay within the dentin (arrow).

tures of extraction sites are summarized below; however, a more detailed description is afforded in the text by Shafer, Hine and Levy.[50]

One-day wound: Fresh blood clot in socket with fibrin on surface; vaso-dilatation of periodontal membrane blood vessels and leucocytic infiltration in area surrounding clot.

Three-day wound: Fibroblast proliferation from periodontal membrane invading clot with peripheral capillary ingrowth. Gingival epithelial proliferation begins. Early osteoclasia of alveolar bone crest begins.

Seven-day wound: Clot becoming well organized by ingrowth of fibro-blasts. Epithelial migration over clot surface may be complete. Early reparative osteoid may be noted.

Fourteen-day wound: Clot almost completely replaced by granulation tissue; young bone trabeculae forming in periphery of socket; wound surface completely epithelialized.

Twenty-one day wound: Continued progressive new bone formation and remodeling restoration of alveolus socket. The process of new bone formation continues until new bone completely fills in the socket.

Extra Teeth

Because of the rare occurrence of extra or supernumerary teeth, this finding is of great significance if encountered in the identification setting. A developmental anomaly, supernumerary teeth are most usually noted between the maxillary central incisors or as maxillary fourth molars (Fig. 36).

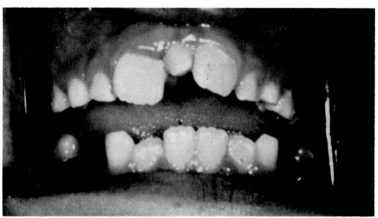

Figure 36. A supernumerary (extra) tooth exists between the two upper central incisors. This condition is rare and bears great specificity. AFIP Neg. No. 58-12725-4.

Restorations and Prostheses

In accordance with the subject matter presented in Chapter II, tooth number or location, surfaces involved, the dental material employed (amalgam, silicate, gold filling, crown, bridge, partial denture) and the restoration outline should be noted. When confronted with bridgework, the abutment teeth and their construction (e.g. full gold crown with plastic facing) as well as the pontic sections (by tooth replacement number and type of construction) should be designated. When dealing with partial dentures, the overall construction as to type of material (pink plastic and/or gold or stainless metals), the number of prosthetic teeth and the natural teeth which serve as the areas of attachment by means of hooks and clasps should be noted.

Decay (Dental Caries)

Decay should be designated by tooth surface and configuration. The appearance of decay varies from small dark-discolored pit-like defects to large areas of cavitation. The smaller lesions may be best demonstrated by a *catch* with the hook explorer. Because of the fact that initially depicted caries on the dentist's tooth chart or an antemortem X ray may have been subsequently removed and replaced by a restoration as found in the postmortem specimen, reference must be made to the *treatment performed* area of the chart to clarify such findings which do not, therefore, represent incompatibilities. It is important to consider the time at which X rays were taken. The primary function of the dental X ray is the demonstration of grossly unobservable carious activity, especially interproximal defects which are not visible upon naked-eye examination. Such affected teeth when discovered, of course, are subsequently restored or extracted. Naturally, only a more recent X ray would reveal subsequent changes. For this reason the most recent X rays will provide a less confusing and more accurate up-to-date evaluation for purposes of comparison (Fig. 37).

Carious areas may lead to fractured teeth on the basis of undermining of the enamel shell. Such fractures are characterized by adjacent irregular noticeable brown discolored decay and are most commonly noted in posterior teeth. In contrast, recent traumatic fractures are most frequently seen in anterior teeth and will disclose an absence of adjacent caries and tend to possess a rather sharp line of fracture edge. With time, antemortem fracture sites become stained by foodstuffs, cigarette tars, etc. although specific aging of the fracture cannot be made. In fractures involving the deeper layers of dentin, the finding of secondary reparative dentin within

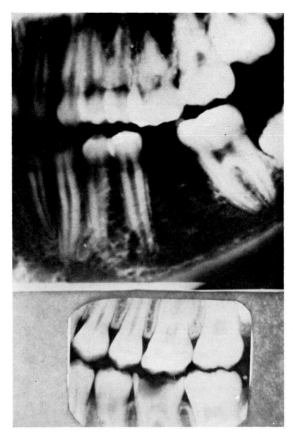

Figure 37. Comparison of postmortem (top) and antemortem (bottom) X ray of the same individual. The carious right lower first molar on the antemortem X ray was extracted leaving the space seen in the postmortem X ray. The *treatment performed* area of the chart indicated that subsequent to the antemortem X ray, tooth 30 was extracted and tooth 29 received two separate occlusal amalgam restorations.

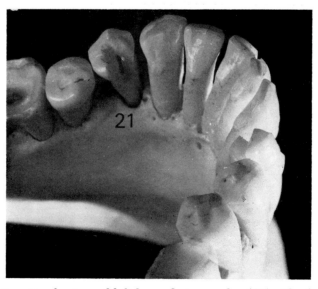

Figure 38. Postmortem fracture of left lower first premolar (21). The fracture extends into the central pulp chamber, and the fracture edges are sharp and unstained. Photograph by P. Besant-Matthews, M.D.

the pulp chamber on histologic section will indicate that the fracture was not recent. Fractures occurring postmortem are frequently noted in teeth of skeletons. This is due to the fact that such teeth become dessicated and brittle and commonly will reveal a loss of enamel due to fracture at the junction of dentin and enamel. Such fractures may also involve both enamel and dentin in which case the line of fracture tends to parallel the long axis of the tooth. Postmortem fracture sites are sharp, clean and unstained (Fig. 38).

Malposition and Malrotation

Malposition refers to crowding, overlapping and spacing abnormalities of individual teeth (Figs. 39 and 40). Malrotation applies to a tooth which is in its expected anatomic arch position but is rotated so that the mesial

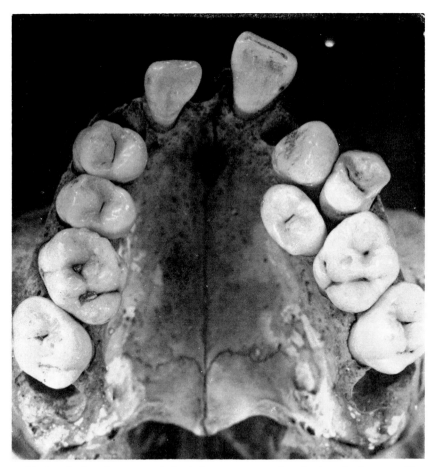

Figure 39. Marked malposition of the left upper premolar. Such a finding would represent an excellent specific feature if related to a bite mark case (discussed in Chap. IX). AFIP Neg. No. 65-1052-8.

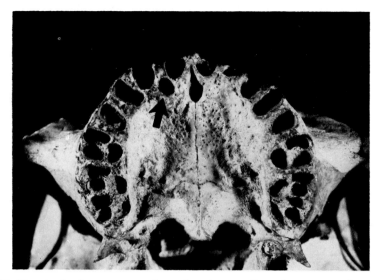

Figure 40. Despite total postmortem loss of entire maxillary dentition in this mongoloid (note parabolic arch curvature) skull, one can state that the right lateral incisor (arrow) was in lingual malposition during life. Such a finding, despite the absence of teeth, may enable specific identification in corroboration with the skeletal determination of race, sex, age and stature.

aspect, for example, may be in the lingual position. The tooth surfaces are designated according to the normal anatomic position of the tooth and not the position indicated by the rotation. Malposition and malrotation of the anterior teeth offer excellent points of comparison in bite mark cases (see Chap. IX). Such changes, however, are not commonly recorded during routine dental examinations and thus should not be considered as inconsistencies in any identification comparison. Antemortem dental casts or X rays will readily disclose the presence of malposition or malrotation.

Peculiar Shapes of Teeth

Alterations in the normal anatomic configuration of a tooth may represent a congenital or acquired condition. The most common congenitally malformed teeth are the Hutchinson incisors of congenital syphilis (Fig. 41) or peg-shaped lateral incisors. These conditions represent rare findings so that they are rather specific characteristics. The former is even less common today in the face of advanced prenatal care in this country.

Acquired changes in tooth shape apply to occupational and habit-induced wear of the teeth structure. Such changes are described below in the discussion of occupational and social changes of the dentition.

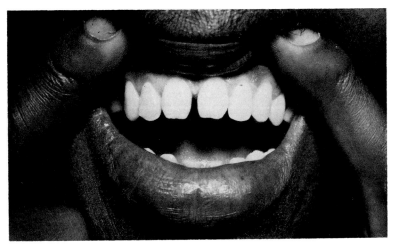

Figure 41. Hutchinson central incisors of congenital syphilis. Note the tapered screwdriver contour. AFIP Neg. No. AMH-8808.

Root Canal Therapy (Endodontia)

As mentioned in Chapter II, such therapy is performed to preserve a tooth which contains a devitalized pulp as a result of caries or trauma. Necrotic pulpal tissue represents a potential focus of local abscess formation and bacteremia and should be removed. This may be accomplished by tooth extraction or, as an expensive alternative, by the mechanical and chemical removal and cleansing of the pulp chamber. The latter procedure represents endodontic therapy and results in the placement of a metallic or cement-like rod or cone within the pulp chamber. Such treatment is immediately conspicuous on the dental X ray and is specific in that it is not a common procedure. It represents expensive dental care. The X ray of such teeth (see Figs. 8 and 9) may disclose not only the rod or cone but also imperfections of the root canal due to instrumentation. On occasion, the root canal cone may even protrude from the apical foramen, representing yet another feature since such an overfill is not the recommended treatment (see Fig. 8). Teeth having had root canal treatment will usually have a full crown visible on naked-eye examination as is indicated by the fact that devitalized teeth become brittle and may subsequently fracture.

Bone Pattern

The spongy bone of the jaws may possess a characteristic persistent X-ray pattern which can be duplicated on the postmortem X ray. In addition, tooth angulation, interproximal space bone loss due to periodontitis and specific changes in pulpal chamber and pulp canal outlines may be present (Figs. 42A and B).

Forensic Dentistry

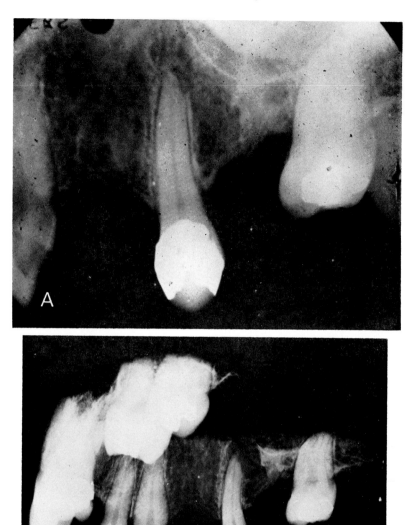

Figure 42. A. Antemortem right posterior maxillary X ray revealing spongy bone pattern between the premolar and molar. B. Postmortem X ray of resected maxilla of same individual showing exact duplication of bone pattern between premolar and molar. Also note the duplication of curvature and slope of the premolar on both X rays.

Complete Dentures

To the untrained eye, complete or full dentures may appear alike in every case. Such is not the truth. Not only may the pink plastic (acrylic) base of the denture possess characterization, but the individual teeth can be of plastic or porcelain in innumerable shapes, sizes and configurations. A dentist or well-trained dental technician may be able to recognize these specific features and should be consulted as to possible clues to identification in such cases. The antemortem records of the dentist who constructed the denture will usually retain a notation as to the material and tooth characteristics for comparison. A previous repair of a broken denture tooth or of the denture itself may be evident and also on record. Some denture teeth may contain pseudo-restoration gold crowns to appear more natural.

Today it is uncommon for the younger general practitioner of dentistry to actually construct a denture with his own hands. (Most general practitioners take the jaw ridge impressions and send them to a commercial dental laboratory for denture construction.) On the other hand, the prosthodontist (denture specialist) or an older practitioner may construct the denture in his own laboratory and may incorporate certain personally recognizable features into the denture. These dentists often can recognize their work at a glance, much like other artisans with their handicrafts. The following case relates such an event:

> In the course of draining a local reservoir, a 1949 Nash automobile containing a human skeleton was discovered settled within the muddy silt of the lake bed. An elderly gentleman, upon seeing the photo of the scene in a newspaper, recognized the car and license plate as belonging to his missing brother who mysteriously disappeared twenty years earlier. Fortunately, the attending dentist, a very close personal friend of the putative deceased, was alive and located. This older dentist specialized in the construction of dentures and had personally made the denture in question in his own laboratory. Despite the fact that the records of the missing man had been destroyed many years ago, the dentist was able to draw and describe the exact details of the prosthetic device. The partial denture was recovered several days later in the muddy lake bed, exactly matched the previous description given by the dentist and was subsequently also identified by him.

For the dentist reader, Haines[18] and Harmeling, et al.[17] elucidate many features of individuality noted in denture construction including

1. shape of palatal relief area;
2. shape and depth of post-dams;
3. labial flange design;
4. retromolar pad coverage;
5. acrylic color and characterization (plain, clear, stippled);

6. tooth shape, size and material; and

7. arch and ridge size.

The denture, of course, should be removed from the mouth and examined on all surfaces. One may surprisingly find a name or identifying number incorporated within the denture base which will lead to rapid identification (Fig. 43). Such denture marking, if standardized, would represent a large step forward in denture identification.[51] Jerman[52] describes details regarding the insertion of a metallic identifying number into the denture while curing.

The author vividly recalls a case in which the police had aptly noted that an unidentified body possessed full dentures; however, they failed to remove the dentures from the mouth. After a fruitless week of search to establish identification, the author was asked to see the case. Identification was promptly made upon removal of the denture which incorporated the social security number of the deceased in the base of the denture.

Although it is rare that one person's denture will properly fit the jaw of another, one may encounter a derelict who may possess the marked denture of another individual. The author has heard of several such instances.

Dentures made for state hospital patients or penitentiary inmates and some armed services laboratories or veterans hospitals may incorporate denture-identifying data. To be totally effective, such a marking system should

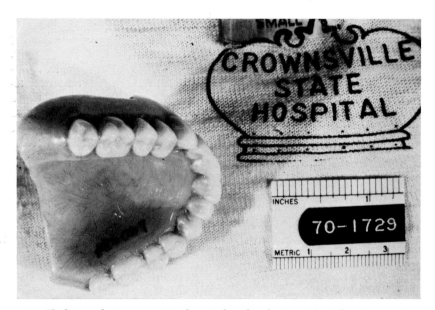

Figure 43. Clothing relating to a state hospital and a denture identification number from that facility established identification in this case.

be standardized (and required by law). While the wearer's initials or a laboratory number may be confirmatory if a putative identity is known, such data is worthless without a suspected identity. The author has encountered several examples of dentures which contained a laboratory identification number; however, without a putative identity, one could never find the laboratory in question to establish the identity. There is no central registry for such information as is available for laundry mark symbols, e.g. In this country, denture incorporation of the social security number would be ideal.

Relationship of the Bite

The observation here concerns the relationship of the teeth of the respective jaws when closed. Specifically, a notation should be made as to whether the upper or lower jaw protrudes upon jaw closure.

Oral Pathology

Deviations in the normal anatomic configurations of the oral structures apply not only to the dentition but also to the oral soft tissues or bone structure and to tongue lesions as well. Although specific pathologic conditions of the oral soft structures are not common, this very fact imparts varying degrees of specificity to the finding depending upon the observed condition. Only commonly encountered findings will be mentioned below.

Mandibular or palatine tori are benign bony excrescences which protrude into the oral cavities. In nonskeletonized remains, such focal exostoses are, of course, covered by oral mucosa. Mandibular tori are generally bilateral (unilateral in about 20% of cases) and are positioned on the lingual side of the mandible in the region of the premolar teeth. The reported incidence in this country is 6 to 8 percent, without any sex difference (Fig. 44). Palatine tori, positioned in the midline of the palate, have been noted in 20 to 35 percent of our population with a female predilection of two to one[53] (Fig. 45). The discovery of tori can be especially helpful in disaster identification situations where the finding may serve as an important differential feature. The condition will usually be noted in antemortem records, although this may not be true for small lesions.

Common tongue abnormalities include geographic tongue, black hairy tongue or scrotal tongue and are conditions which may be noted by family members (Fig. 46).

The finding of Dilantin®-induced hyperplasia of the gums may not only serve as an identification aid but may also suggest the cause of death: namely, epileptic seizure. The pathologist should examine the tongue for lacerations or contusions in such cases. Chronic heavy metal poisoning,

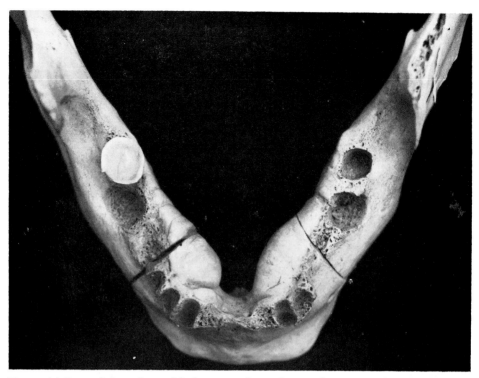

Figure 44. Large bilateral mandibular tori in lingual premolar regions (oblique sawcuts are artefact). The remaining molar on the right shows marked attritional wear of the occlusal surface, suggesting a very elderly individual.

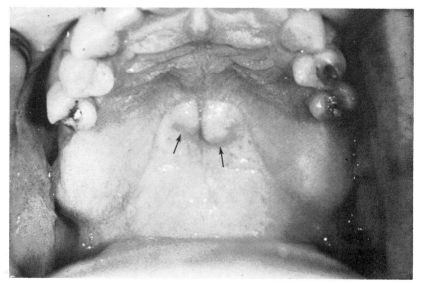

Figure 45. Palatine torus in usual midline location (arrows). AFIP Neg. No. 58-12725-6.

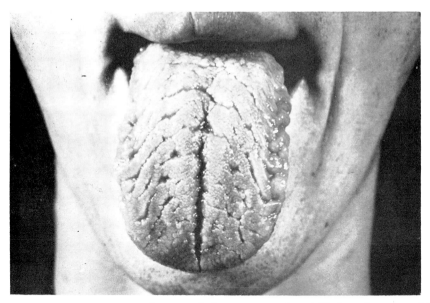

Figure 46. Scrotal tongue; so designated due to unusual wrinkled surface resembling skin of the scrotum. Abnormalities of the tongue are unusual and therefore bear high degrees of specificity.

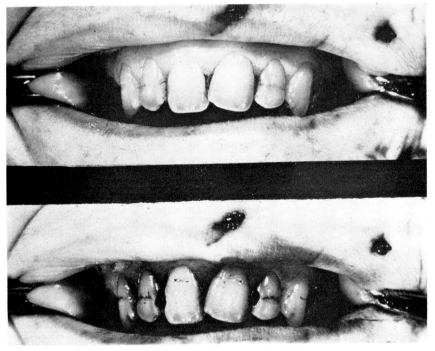

Figure 47. Horizontal linear pitting of the labial surfaces of the upper anterior teeth. The bottom half of the figure shows the degree to which such irregularities can be delineated by the application of a dye (such as gentian violet) to the teeth.

such as lead poisoning, may cause pigmentation of the gums and thereby suggest a cause of death or may represent a clue as to the occupation of the deceased.

The commonly seen linear pitted defects in the enamel structure of the anterior teeth may relate to febrile illnesses during childhood and may prove to be a corroborative feature in identification (Fig. 47).

Any known preexisting bone pathology, such as cysts of dental or bone origin, can be revealed by postmortem radiography for comparison with available antemortem X rays.

The following case discloses the value of a rare pathologic finding, namely, a healed oro-antral fistula as a complication of a previous upper molar extraction, in the identification of a burned body:

On a cold winter evening a fire occurred in an abandoned downtown Baltimore warehouse which was a known habitat for homeless, wandering alcoholics. The Arson Squad discovered the charred body of a white male within the ruins. The dental structures of the deceased were intact; however, a period of five weeks elapsed before a lead developed which eventually solved the identity. The wife of the deceased had heard from a local *wino* that her husband had died in the above incident. She contacted the Medical Examiner's Office where the autopsy was performed and stated her husband had received care at a local state hospital. She also said that as a result of such treatment he had suffered a peculiar condition wherein every time he blew his nose, *air would whistle through an opening in his upper jaw*. The upper jaw was then dissected, and a healed oro-antral fistula of the right posterior maxillary region was noted. The state hospital dental records later confirmed this and other points of comparison (Fig. 48).

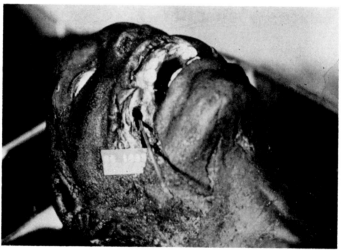

Figure 48. Probe inserted into oro-antral fistula of charred body.

Occupational Changes and Socioeconomic Patterns of the Dentition

Certain occupations or personal habits may induce unusual wear or attritional patterns in the dentition. The habitual opening of bobby pins (as in females or male hairdressers) with the anterior teeth may result in a notching of the incisal aspect of the upper central incisors. Carpenters, shoemakers, upholsterers, seamstresses and tailors may similarly develop notching of the central incisors from holding nails or pins. Workers exposed to abrasive dust (e.g. sandblasters, etc.) may develop more generalized attritional alteration of the dentition. Certain musicians may develop broad attritional changes of the anterior teeth due to clenching of the instrument mouthpiece. Inveterate pipe smokers (or even cigar smokers with bite stems) also develop broad areas of excessive wear generally located in the lateral incisor, cuspid or premolar regions (Fig. 49).

The socioeconomic status of the deceased may be suggested by the nature and characteristics of the observed dental care. The presence of multiple crowns, bridgework, gold restorations and root canal therapy all bear the connotation of a generally well-educated individual of more than modest income standards. In contrast, the presence of poor oral hygiene characterized by few restorations, many decayed teeth and signs of periodontitis (inflammation of the gums) generally designate an individual

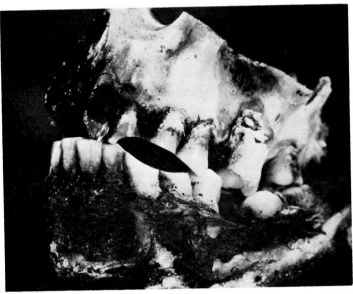

Figure 49. Typical pipe smoker's wear of teeth. This finding conclusively identified a burned body for which a putative identity was established on the basis of the circumstances surrounding death and a nonspecific wristwatch.

of low socioeconomic status. In addition, the finding of many previously extracted teeth without replacement by bridgework or partial dentures also correlates with persons of lower social strata.

There are also certain geographic differences in the use and design of various restorative techniques and materials. This fact may be of value in differentiation of mass disaster victims. Geographic differences in dental methods and material do not exist in native U.S. citizens, but such differences have been of value in several European air crash disasters wherein the victims were of varied national origins.[54, 55]

The following identification case cites an example wherein the nature and idiosyncrasies of the dental work suggested the location where the work was performed:

A human skeleton containing a .38 caliber missile, numerous shotgun pellets and several fractured ribs was found in an isolated wooded area of Baltimore. Death was believed due to a shotgun wound of the chest. The dentition was recovered intact. Dental examination disclosed several restorations, many of which were of gold foil material. In addition, evidence of a left mandibular abscess was noted upon examination of the jaws (Fig. 50). The neatness of the restorations in general and especially the presence of gold foil as a filling material strongly suggested that the work may have been performed at a dental school, more specifically, the local University of Maryland School of Dentistry. (Gold foil is a superior restorative material but is expensive and extremely time-consuming to insert. It is generally found in two populations: in the well-to-do person who

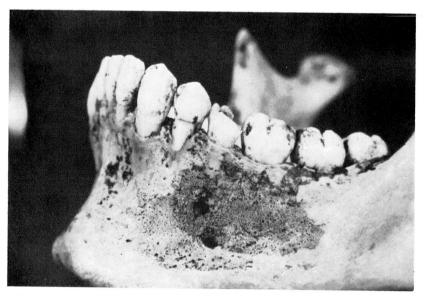

Figure 50. An abscess perforation of the outer plate of the mandible is present adjacent to the root apex of the second premolar. The surrounding discolored pitted surface of the bone indicates antemortem periostitis due to the abscess.

can afford the care and in the indigent where the work is obtained in dental schools, thus enabling dental students to gain skills in the handling of gold foil material). To establish identification we were prepared to examine the dental school patient records of all Negro males from ages eighteen to twenty-six, the latter figures suggested by anthropological data retrieved from the skeleton. Fortunately, we were spared such a search, for at this time the wife of the deceased, having read about the finding of the skeleton in a newspaper, reminded police of an earlier report regarding her missing husband filed three months previously. Interrogation of his wife revealed that her husband had received treatment at the dental school and had complained of a sore lower jaw with extreme swelling when last seen three months earlier. The dental school records under the husband's name disclosed a perfect comparison with the skeletal findings.

Race and Sex Determination from the Teeth

This topic is mentioned to caution the reader that race and sex determination based upon the dentition is extremely hazardous. The total skeletal survey is considerably more accurate than the teeth in such determinations. It is best to consult an anthropologist if faced with race and sex analysis from the dentition alone. The variability in tooth and arch characteristics regarding these parameters frequently results in unreliable conclusions. Lasker and Lee[56] as well as Aitchison[57] present data regarding racial features of the dentition.

In consideration of sex determination among preadolescent children, Hunt and Gleiser[58] have established data indicating that close agreement of hand bone age and dental age is indicative of a male whereas divergence between hand bone age and dental age is indicative of a female.

THE CONCLUSIONS OF THE COMPARISON OF ANTEMORTEM AND POSTMORTEM FINDINGS

The reader will recall that *comparison equals identification*. The author has also mentioned that the more alterations or abnormalities that exist in a given mouth, the greater are the points for potential comparison which serve in establishing a positive identification. The important feature of dental identification is that a positive comparison must bear no incompatibilities and any inconsistencies must be adequately explained to effect a perfect match between the antemortem and postmortem data. One cannot state, as a generalization, that *x* number of points of comparison must exist before a positive identification can be established. One must realize that the total circumstances of the identification situation must be considered and that only a single tooth or jaw fragment may possess the degree of specificity necessary to establish positive identification. The latter comment especially applies to a comparison of radiographs (Figs. 51 and 52). The final decision as to correctness or degree of credibility of the identifi-

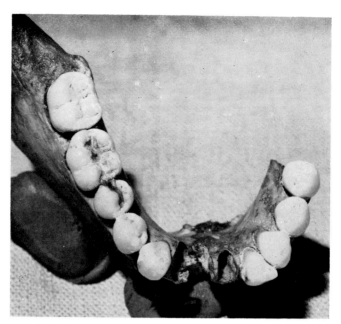

Figure 51. A mandible fragment with an MO amalgam of the first molar and a DO amalgam of the second premolar. Although the naked-eye findings were consistent with the putative identity, this particular combination of restorations is common; therefore, the conclusion is derived that the skeleton is consistent with the putative identity but not necessarily specific for that individual alone.

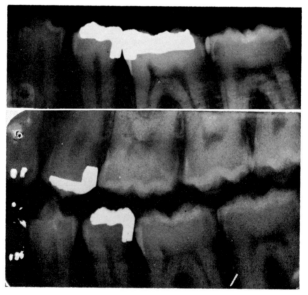

Figure 52. However, a postmortem X ray (top) of the Figure 51 jawbone, when compared with the antemortem X ray of the putative identity (bottom), discloses an exact comparison in the morphology of the DO amalgam of the premolar. The X ray comparison thereby elevates the dental data from *consistent* to *specific*. The molar filling in the postmortem X ray, of course, was placed subsequent to the first X ray and was so indicated in the treatment section of the records.

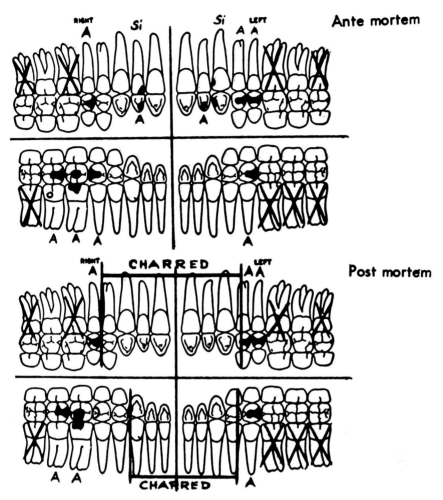

Figure 53. Antemortem (top) and postmortem (bottom) dental record comparison of charred body shows that despite total loss of the anterior dentition, more than enough points of comparison without inconsistencies remain to establish identification. Note the matching extracted teeth (crossed out) and the restoration surfaces and morphology.

cation rests within the judgment and experience of the identification expert upon consideration of all the elements and data applicable to the situation.

To further elaborate, a positive comparison based upon one or several teeth can lead to positive identification provided the comparable findings match for only the one unidentified body within a known set of putative identities. That is to say that if a comparable set of nonspecific restoration patterns pertain to only one body within a closed population (as in an air crash setting), then positive identification can be established (Figs. 53 and 54A and B).

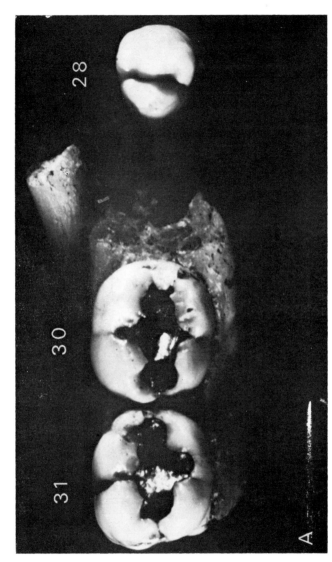

Figure 54A. Fragment of the right lower jaw containing teeth 30, 31 and a separately recovered 28. The second premolar (29) was not recovered postmortem. Teeth 30 and 31 each possess single surface occlusal amalgam restorations, as seen. The first premolar (28) is restoration-free.

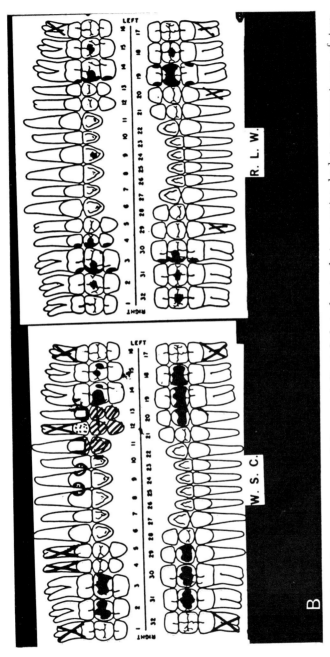

Figure 54B. The circumstances of the case indicated that the teeth in question had to represent one of two people, either W.S.C. or R.L.W. Antemortem records for each indicated W.S.C. This identification is primarily based on the fact that tooth 30 for R. L. W. is a two-surfaced DO filling. Based upon the naked-eye findings of these three teeth alone, one cannot establish absolute identification for W.S.C. to exclusion of others; however, with only two possiblities the identity of W.S.C. was absolutely established.

On the other hand, given a comparable set of nonspecific restoration patterns of one or several teeth without the exclusion of the population at large, the expert is left with the opinion that the postmortem findings are *consistent with* but not *specific for* the putative identity in question. The final placement of such a case with few teeth for assay into a *consistent* or *specific* category will depend upon the specificity inherent to the particular findings and upon the judgment of the investigator. The value of X-ray comparison is most appreciated in such an instance. The X ray may serve to greatly increase the specificity value of the naked-eye findings and, hence, enable a positive identification specific for that one person to the exclusion of any other possibilities (Figs. 51 and 52).

The fact that the dental identification procedure may result in only a *consistent* conclusion may in itself be a significant contribution. One must remember that the dental comparison will be utilized in collation with other modes of identification or with the circumstances of disappearance to elevate the credibility of the identification (see Chaps. III and IV).

The above discussion further emphasizes the importance of the postmortem recovery of as many dental structures as possible. A return visit to the site of body discovery may be necessary in an attempt to locate a specific tooth. The examiner should also consider postmortem head and neck X rays to locate dislodged teeth in the hypopharynx or even the X-ray examination of dirt or charred debris if necessary.

Chapter VIII

THE DETERMINATION OF CHRONOLOGICAL AGE BY THE DENTITION

GENERAL CONSIDERATIONS

O N OCCASION, the assessment of the chronological age of human remains by the dentition may represent a critical aspect of the body identification. Before specifically discussing age determination from the teeth, it is necessary to present the overall approach by the forensic pathologist to age determination of the unidentified human body. A variety of observations provide data for age estimation; however, the dentition, especially in earlier years, and the skeleton serve as the primary scientific methods for age estimation.

Initial observations about age include the nature of any clothing or personal effects present with the remains. Such items, especially in a mass disaster setting, may provide superficial clues to the age range of the deceased, that is, youth, early adulthood, middle age and old age. The subsequent autopsy examination provides a more scientific method of age estimation. It must be appreciated that concomitant with aging, body tissues undergo alterations detectable by naked-eye and microscopic examination. Specifically, the degree of atherosclerosis of the coronary arteries and aorta, the morphology of the prostate gland and internal female genitalia, and the presence or absence of certain pathologic conditions within the kidneys and lungs provide information enabling a crude estimation of age range to be established. If more precision regarding age is required, in general terms, the skeleton must provide the necessary data.

When dealing with skeletonized remains, age estimation of the skeleton is a primary objective of such an examination. Even in the case of a more complete human body, of course, the skeletal structures may still be bared for specific areas of interest. The reference here is to the easily removed and cleaned symphysis pubis.

Examination of the skeleton relevant to age determination centers upon numerous anatomical areas. The inherent value of age estimation from the bones is due to the fact that until the early twenties one may observe

113

the processes of bone growth and maturation; in later years, aging changes of the fully formed bone structures may be recognized. In early childhood the status of development of the hand bones provides a reliable indicator of chronologic age. Throughout the teens the status of epiphyseal closure of the long bones serves as the anthropologic means of age estimation. Through the late teens and early twenties, the status of closure of the vertebral and pelvic bones are utilized as age indicators. The morphologic changes in the face of the symphysis pubis, the status of skull suture closure and subsequent aging changes of the skeleton in general provide the criteria for age estimation from the twenties and beyond. Although many forensic pathologists possess basic introductory knowledge about the total aspects of skeletal examination (this includes age, race, sex and stature determination), if such an examination is critical, a physical anthropologist should be consulted. The anthropologist can reliably estimate age from skeletal structures within a range of plus or minus one year to plus or minus eight years; the latter figure applies to the more elderly population, the former to the child skeleton. Kerley[8] has also devised a method whereby microscopic sections of long bones can be used for age determination. For specific details regarding the totality of skeletal examination, the reader is referred to Krogman's excellent text on the subject.[59]

It is toward the above overview of age determination of unknown remains that the dental examination turns to provide further data for the investigator. It should be noted that the teeth represent the most reliable indicator of chronologic age from birth to fourteen years. Such measurements, of course, are derived from the fact that during this period of life there is continued development and intermixture of the primary dental follicle through the progressive stages of tooth calcification terminating in mature root development with closure of the apical foramen. During this period of birth to fourteen years, utilization of the various methods to be described below are considered reliable within approximately one year more or less. Dental development during this period possesses a lesser degree of variability as compared with other maturational events such as skeletal development.[60] Beyond the age of fourteen years, dental age estimation based upon the naked-eye and radiographic examination of second and third molar development and upon current knowledge is less precise. Beyond the early twenties, following completion of the development of the third molar, dental age estimation becomes but a crude criterion for age estimation of remains unless specialized histologic methods are employed as discussed below.

The estimation of age from the teeth can be performed utilizing naked-eye observation of the emergence pattern or attritional change, radiographic methods or histologic techniques. Estimation of chronologic age based upon emergence patterns or attritional wear of the dentition is less precise compared to the use of radiographic or histologic techniques. This statement especially applies to the criterion of attrition as a valid indicator of chronologic age. The reason for this is obvious; coarseness of diet is a primary factor in dental attrition. This is a well-known fact and has fostered the statement, "Don't look a gift horse in the mouth" to thereby evaluate the age of the animal and, thus, the value of the gift. The author has seen numerous young skulls of nineteenth-century American Indians as well as of modern mongoloid Vietnamese, and the degree of dental attrition is striking when compared with similar age and attritional patterns of the current American population. One must realize that an estimation of age by dental attrition is quite crude; and certainly, an age estimation by total skeletal examination serves as a far more accurate chronologic indicator. In a similar context an evaluation of age based upon the degree of periodontal disease, interdental bone resorption and apical migration of the gingival attachment also provides but a crude estimate.

The use of the emergence sequence of the developing dentition to estimate age also reveals considerable variability and is less exact than radiographic analysis of the jaw structures. The emergence sequence refers to the eruption status of those teeth noted to have penetrated the gingiva and does not consider the total developmental status of the jaws in question as does the radiograph. Hurme[61, 62] has provided extensive data on the emergence sequence of the permanent dentition based upon 100,000 children. Falkner[63] presents data on the eruption patterns of the deciduous dentition as derived from a longitudinal study of approximately 200 children ranging in age from four weeks to three years. His data provides the total number of erupted teeth present at varying age plateaus in the four-week to three-year range.

Although the emergence pattern alone may be useful in certain identification situations, if a more accurate age estimate is indicated one must utilize the radiograph which will provide additional information concerning the totality of crown and root development of the unerupted dentition. In essence, tooth emergence represents but one phase of tooth development; with a slightly greater expenditure of time, much more accurate data is derived from the taking of a radiograph which will disclose a panorama of tooth development.

Specific information concerning radiologic and histologic methods for age estimation are discussed below.

DENTAL AGE ESTIMATION OF THE FETUS OR THE YOUNG INFANT

The histologic examination of the jaw structures of the fetus provide information regarding intrauterine age. Kraus[64] has studied a series of ninety-five human fetuses ranging in age from eight to eighteen weeks. His histologic examination disclosed that the deciduous teeth (the central incisors) begin calcification as early as twelve weeks or as late as sixteen weeks. The remaining deciduous teeth follow in regular sequence from the central incisor to the second molar.

Stack[65] established data concerning prenatal and postnatal dental age spanning the interval from the seventh intrauterine month to seven months after birth. The method concerns a sum of the dissected total dry tooth weights as compared to known gestation or postnatal age.

Boyde[66] and Miles[67] have both investigated the use of histologic ground sections of teeth to arrive at chronologic age based upon the degree of enamel and dentin formation adjacent to the neonatal line, the histologic marker of the time of birth.

The composite chart of dental development devised by Gustafson[68] and Koch, to be discussed further below, also depicts the intrauterine stages of beginning mineralization and the stages of postnatal crown completion of the deciduous dentition.

DENTAL AGE ESTIMATION FROM BIRTH TO TWENTY YEARS

From birth until approximately fourteen years, the developmental patterns and eruption schedules of the deciduous teeth, followed by the ensuing intermixture of the development and eruption of the permanent dentition, serve as the most reliable indicators of chronologic age (Fig. 55). From the ages of fourteen to twenty-three years, the residual growth of the second molar root structures and the third molar development through apical closure represent a means of chronologic age estimation; however, there is greater variability in these parameters than exists during the earlier years of dental development. In the fourteen to twenty-three year range, the skeletal structures rate superior to the teeth in relation to chronologic age estimation.

The works of Hurme[61, 62] and Falkner[63] regarding eruption (emergence) patterns in children only have been mentioned earlier under "General Considerations."

One of the earliest studies regarding the chronology of tooth development is that performed by Massler and Schour.[69] Their data is based upon observations of thirty infants' and children's jaws, many of whom were debilitated, from the ages of five months *in utero* to fifteen years. The

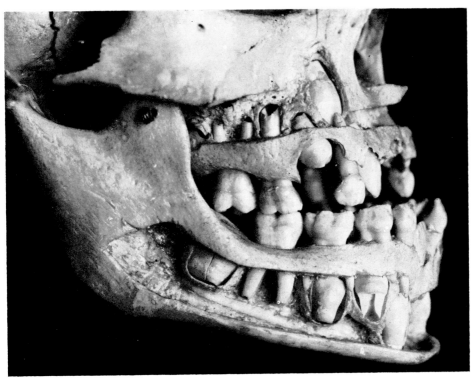

Figure 55. Dissection of jaw structures indicating intermixture of primary and secondary dentitions. The estimated age of the remains, as compared with the Schour-Massler data (Figs. 56 and 57), is 7.5 years. Photograph by P. Besant-Matthews, M.D.

small number and the health status of this sample population has resulted in some criticism of the data; however, Miles[70] states that the Schour-Massler data appears to give useful and reliable results. Specifically, the works of Brauer and Badahur[71]; Garn, Lewis and Polacheck[72]; and Moorrees, Fanning and Hunt[73] all indicate a greater range in variability of tooth development than that noted in the Schour and Massler data. The Schour-Massler charts on tooth development are simple to use for direct comparison with postmortem radiographs and are illustrated in Figures 56 and 57. Table V presents a chronologic chart of the dentition based upon the Schour-Massler data.

Moorrees, Fanning and Hunt[73] have presented an extensive longitudinal study of the development of ten permanent teeth, specifically the maxillary incisors and the eight teeth of the mandibular quadrant. Their data presents the age of attainment for fourteen arbitrarily selected stages of tooth formation beginning with the initial phase of crown development

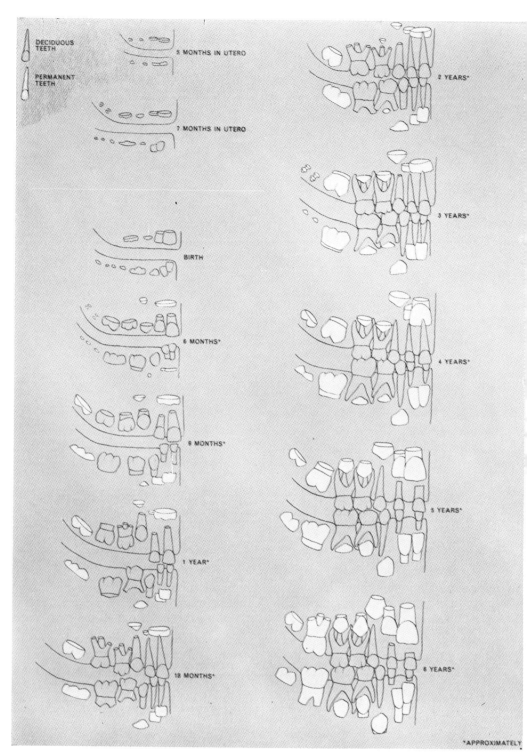

Figure 56. The Schour-Massler Development Chart from birth until six years. Courtesy of Morrey and Nelsen, *Dental Science Handbook*.

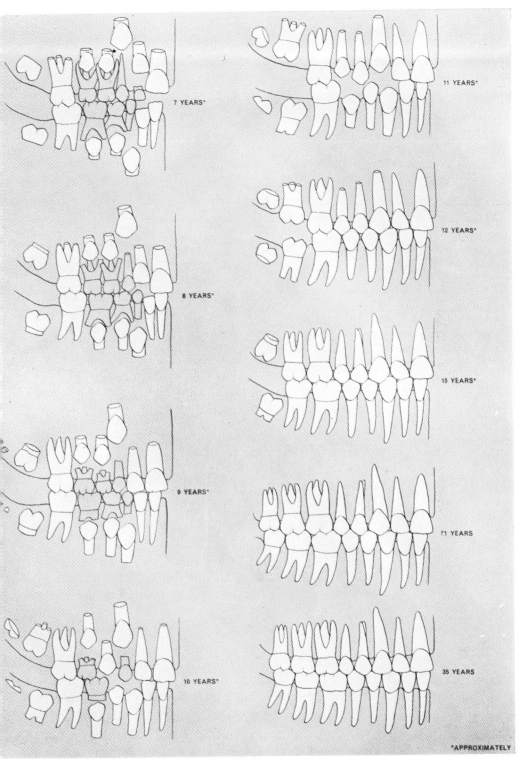

Figure 57. The Schour-Massler Development Chart from seven years to maturity. Courtesy of Morrey and Nelsen, *Dental Science Handbook*.

TABLE V

CHRONOLOGY OF THE HUMAN DENTITION*

Tooth	Maxillary Eruption	Maxillary R.C.†	Mandibular Eruption	Mandibular R.C.†
Deciduous dentition *(baby teeth)*				
Central incisor	7½ mo.	1½ yr.	6 mo.	1½ yr.
Lateral incisor	9 mo.	2 yr.	7 mo.	1½ yr.
Cuspid (canine)	18 mo.	3¼ yr.	16 mo.	3¼ yr.
First molar	14 mo.	2½ yr.	12 mo.	2¼ yr.
Second molar	24 mo.	3 yr.	20 mo.	3 yr.
Permanent dentition				
Central incisor	7-8 yr.	10 yr.	6-7 yr.	9 yr.
Lateral incisor	8-9 yr.	11 yr.	7-8 yr.	10 yr.
Cuspid (canine)	11-12 yr.	13-15 yr.	9-10 yr.	12-14 yr.
First premolar	10-11 yr.	12-13 yr.	10-12 yr.	12-13 yr.
Second premolar	10-12 yr.	12-14 yr.	11-12 yr.	13-14 yr.
First molar	6-7 yr.	9-10 yr.	6-7 yr.	9-10 yr.
Second molar	12-13 yr.	14-16 yr.	11-13 yr.	14-15 yr.
Third molar	17-21 yr.	18-25 yr.	17-21 yr.	18-25 yr.

* From Logan, W. H. and Kronfeld, R.; slightly modified by McCall, J. O. and Schour, I., *Journal of the American Dental Association,* 23:139 (1936).
† Root completed; X-ray examination necessary.

through closure of the apical foramen. The study was based upon the dental formation of 336 subjects followed by serial radiographic examination so that precise levels of attainment of crown and root development as compared with chronologic age could be established. The data is presented in excellent monogram style according to sex and particular tooth. Furthermore, the range of variability in age for each stage of tooth formation is included. The charts are easy to use and a practical example of their application is provided. This data provides more precise age estimations when compared to the less comprehensive study of Massler and Schour noted above.

Fanning,[74] in an earlier study, also provides the chronology of the formation of the deciduous mandibular canine and the first and second molars as well as the chronology of the stages of root resorption of the deciduous maxillary incisors and the mandibular quadrant. This excellent work, a longitudinal study, also provides the age variability expressed in percentiles.

Nolla[75] developed a small radiographic study of twenty-five male and twenty-five female subjects from ages two to seventeen years, wherein he plotted chronologic age versus the stage of development of the permanent dentition. The data is more difficult to utilize than the above-described work of Moorrees, Fanning and Hunt since one must rate the stage of tooth development, convert this rating to Nolla's point system and then consult his developmental curves depicting point values and age.

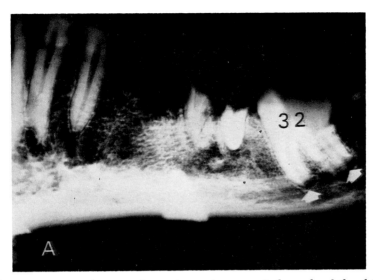

Figure 58A. Note incomplete root formation and open apical canals of the third molar (32). Both skeletal age and dental age indicated an estimated chronologic age of eighteen years.

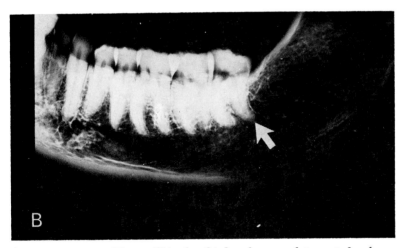

Figure 58B. In contrast to Figure 58A, the third molar complete root development and apical closure indicate an age of more than twenty-two years. More specific determination of age in such a case would depend upon the skeletal findings. AFIP Neg. No. 72-6179-1.

Gustafson[76] and Koch have also compiled data from multiple literature sources and have constructed a concise diagrammatic chart of dental development. Their charting includes the total spectrum of tooth development beginning with intrauterine mineralization of the primary dentition and terminating with the second permanent molar root development at age sixteen. Four different landmarks of tooth formation (beginning of crown mineralization, completion of crown formation, eruption and completion of root formation) for each tooth are plotted against chronologic age. An indication of the variability for each landmark is also provided. The Gustafson and Koch chart is easy to use; however, it is less precise as to chronologic age than the Moorrees, Fanning and Hunt data due to the measurement of tooth formation based upon only four landmarks.

As one approaches the age period beyond fourteen years, age determination based upon tooth development depends primarily on the root development of the second permanent molar and the third molar. With a loss in the multiple foci of developmental data as provided by numerous teeth in earlier years, age determination by the dentition becomes more variable and less precise. The development of the third molar especially reveals, in the writer's experience, a considerable degree of variation; and furthermore, little work has been done comparing third molar development with chronologic age. Miles[67] has stated that the third molar is complete in length with beginning closure of the apical canals by age eighteen years; the apical canals are usually closed by twenty years; at age twenty-two years, the apices are usually closed and constricted (Figs. 58A and B).

DENTAL AGE ESTIMATION BEYOND AGE TWENTY

It should again be emphasized that naked-eye and radiographic examination of the teeth in this age category provides but a crude estimation of true chronologic age (Figs. 59 and 60). A much more reliable estimate of chronologic age is afforded by examination of the skeleton, specifically, the degree of skull suture closure, the status of the symphysis pubis and the total skeletal survey. Attritional change, periodontal status and bone resorption are not specific indicators of age.

In contrast to the above statements, however, the application of histologic examination of ground tooth sections to derive age estimation has proven accurate in the hands of experienced investigators. Such histologic techniques were pioneered by Gustafson.[76] The Gustafson method of age determination based upon histologic examination of tooth ground sections centers upon various changes in the tooth structure dependent upon chronologic aging. The specific criteria observed are attrition, paradentosis, secondary dentin formation, cementum apposition, root resorption and root

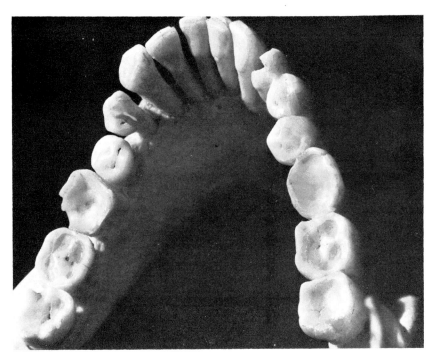

Figure 59. Naked-eye observation of the marked occlusal wear (attrition) of the premolar and molar teeth suggests an elderly person, perhaps sixty years of age or older. Photograph by P. Besant-Matthews, M.D.

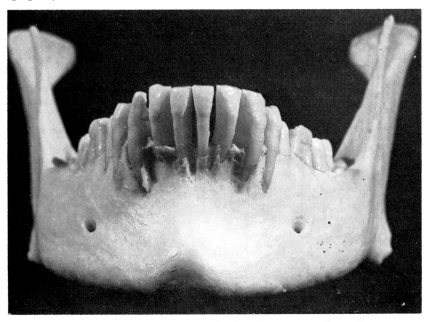

Figure 60. The marked loss of stabilizing alveolar bone surrounding the anterior teeth is another feature generally correlated with a person fifty years of age or older. Such bone loss or attrition (Fig. 59) is a very crude and unreliable indicator of chronologic age. Photograph by P. Besant-Matthews, M.D.

transparency. Gustafson classified each of these six age criteria of teeth of established chronologic age into a grading system based upon four stages indicating the degree of age change per criterion. In this manner, each criterion was awarded a point value depending upon the degree of change as noted upon microscopic examination of the histologic ground sections. The total point sum derived from all six criteria for a particular tooth then formed a regression line plotting point sum versus known chronologic age. In this manner a body of data was collected providing total points as correlated with known chronologic age. Upon application of this technique to teeth of unknown age, Gustafson achieved an average error of plus or minus 3.6 years.

Gustafson's study was based upon a Swedish population. Nalbandian and Sognnaes[77] applied the Gustafson method to a Boston population and an average error of plus or minus 7.9 years was obtained.

The Gustafson method is an extremely academic examination dependent upon subjective interpretation of the various degrees of aging change by competent observers who have studied large numbers of teeth of both known and unknown ages. As with any examination, the reliability of the techniques in the hands of persons not experienced in such evaluations reduces the value of the method when applied to practical forensic dentistry. In view of the latter statement, Miles[70] has stated that ground section examination pertaining to the criterion of root translucency alone might prove to be of some value to the inexperienced examiner.

Chapter IX

BITE MARK ANALYSIS

GENERAL CONSIDERATIONS

BITE MARK COMPARISON represents a vital contribution of dentistry to the forensic sciences. The comparison involves the bite mark pattern at the scene of the crime with the dental alignment and characteristics of the dentition of a suspect. Depending upon the circumstances, bite mark patterns may be deposited within foodstuffs and other objects or upon the victim of an assault or homicide. Bite marks inflicted by a deceased victim upon the living assailant may also be noted.

A point that must be established at this stage of bite mark discussion is that the forensic pathologist is not qualified to handle bite mark analysis since the techniques and data interpretation require the knowledge of the dentist. Even dental experts in the field of bite mark analysis admit to the difficulties inherent in the bite mark comparison.

The responsibilities of the pathologist or criminologist when confronted with a bite mark case are

1. recognition of the injury pattern as being consistent with a bite mark,
2. the immediate notification of a dental consultant,
3. the proper procedure to follow regarding the bitten tissue or substance and
4. the recovery of possible secretory substance from saliva coating the bitten tissue.

In general terms, the bite mark analysis is concerned with a comparison of a life-size photographic reproduction of the bitten area (subject or object) with the dental models of a suspect. (Dental models are made from impressions of the suspect's mouth and are therefore identical to the dentition and are life-size.) Many different methods have been utilized to accomplish such a comparison; however, the common basic concept has been to delineate the pressure-inducing incisal and cuspal surfaces of the suspect's dental models and to record these surfaces in such a manner that they may be superimposed upon the bite mark photograph or qualitatively measured for comparison with similar measurements from the photograph.

Ström[78] credits Sörup as being the first bite mark analyst dating back to 1924. Sörup made varnished dental casts of the suspect, applied printer's ink to the incisal surfaces and transferred the incisal imprint to moistened transparent paper. The transparent paper was then superimposed upon the life-size bite mark photographs to achieve a comparison.

Buhtz and Erhardt[79] attempted to reproduce tissue consistency by placing baker's dough upon sponge rubber around a central pole. Articulated suspect dental models than *bit* the phantom limb, and a diapositive of the tooth impressions in the dough was compared with the actual bite mark photograph.

Morgen[80] made models of both the bite mark and the suspect's dentition. Using black paint he highlighted the tooth indentations on the bite mark model and similarly applied black paint to the suspect's dental models so that only the incisal and occlusal surfaces remained bare. Photographic negatives of both the bite mark and suspect casts were then superimposed, and a comparison was achieved.

Ström[78] articulated the suspect's models, applied fatty lipstick to the incisal surfaces, transferred the incisal areas to transparent paper and then superimposed the transparency upon the bite mark photograph.

Furness[81] introduced a method in 1968 which utilizes enlarged comparison photographs of the bite mark and the suspect's dental casts. The method of presenting the evidence is similar to tool mark and ballistic comparison methods common to forensic scientists. His method is briefly outlined:

1. An enlarged photograph of the bite mark is made.
2. Printer's ink is applied to the incisal aspects of the suspect's models.
3. Photographs of the front (labial) and top (occlusal) views of the casts are made. These photographs are printed to correspond in size with the previous enlarged bite mark photographs.
4. The enlarged photographs of the bite mark and the suspect's models are then mounted adjacent to each other on cardboard, and lines are drawn to indicate similarities.

This method is excellent for presentation of evidence to a lay jury.

The above methods are presented to expose the reader to the basic approach of bite mark analysis. It is important to realize that there exists no single method which must be utilized in bite mark studies. The method used by any particular investigator will depend upon personal preferences and one's ability to handle or accommodate a particular format. The author prefers to utilize photographs and measurements of Aluwax® bites of articulated suspects' models for comparison with the actual bite mark photograph.

Although any surface area of the human body may serve as the focus of a bite mark, the head, neck, breasts and thighs are common areas. The bite lesion may vary in degree of injury from mild skin contusions to avulsion of the bitten part. Several authors[82] have stated that the incidence of bite marks in homicide cases tends to be concentrated within homosexual or heterosexual homicides representing crimes of passion or child abuse. The author might add that the combination of strangulation and/ or blunt force injury, sexual assault and the presence of bite marks tend to form a triad of findings in the heterosexual psychopathic variety of homicide. The term *psychopathic* is included by the author and is not meant to imply that all such cases involve psychopathic killers. The designation of the psychiatric status of an assailant at the time of a crime is reserved for the forensic psychiatrist, not the forensic pathologist, and certainly is not an area of expertise for the dentist.

Upon the discovery of a possible bite mark injury, the pathologist or responsible official investigating the crime should immediately contact the dental consultant to establish a further course of action. This must be done as soon as possible because the necessary examination of the bite mark should be performed prior to any further manipulation of the tissue. The performance of the autopsy and handling of the body prior to the bite mark analysis may cause unnecessary artefactual change of the bite mark and thereby introduce error into the comparison analysis. Immediate action upon bite mark cases is essential because further postmortem change may lead to shrinkage or bloating of tissue, the loss of tooth indentations or the further diffusion of contusion hemorrhage, thus distorting the original tooth pattern. On the other hand, the bite mark should also be reexamined one or two days following the initial injury since indiscriminate, vague contusions or abrasions may show to better advantage after a longer postmortem interval. The forensic pathologist is aware of this delayed appearance phenomenon from his experience with neck abrasions in conjunction with strangulation cases, for example.

The prevention of delay in bite mark examination is best accomplished by the prearranged availability of a dental consultant, preferably one who has had some knowledge of or experience with bite mark analysis. The question of the selection of such a person may arise. The immediate availability of a dentist with bite mark expertise is a rarity. There are only a few dentists throughout the world who possess any experience concerning bite mark analysis. The fact exists, however, that any dentist possesses the knowledge capable of performing such an analysis although it is best if such an individual is associated with a dental teaching center. This preference is stated because the dentist affiliated with a dental school has easy access to the photographic techniques necessary for the examination, has consultation available with other nearby colleagues in the dental specialties if necessary and is probably located in proximity to a dental or medical library where text and journal articles on the subject can be studied. In addition, the dental school staff member is more likely to have the time so necessary to deal with a bite mark problem, since the analysis of suspected assailants and the subsequent medicolegal trial testimony may involve numerous tedious hours, a commodity of which the busy general practitioner has little.

Upon subsequent trial testimony, the question regarding expertise on the part of the dentist handling his first bite mark case may arise. However, the basic facts to remember are that (1) bite mark cases are so rare that only a few persons in the world have handled more than an occasional case and (2) the method of bite mark comparison is scientific and speaks for itself. The majority of the cases in the literature are authored by foreign investigators, and only a scant few dentists who have had any experience in bite mark analysis in this country are known to this author.

On occasion, one is confronted with the finding of nonhuman bite injuries upon the deceased. Animal bites are usually easily distinguished from human bite injuries due to differences in arch alignment and specific tooth morphology. Dog bites, perhaps the most common nonhuman bite, are characterized by a narrow anterior dental arch and consist of deep tooth wounds over a small area. The dog has small central and broad lateral incisors compared with the broad central and narrow lateral incisors of the human. The dog (or other carnivorous mammal) is more apt to cause avulsion of human tissue during violent biting than is the human, although portions of breasts or ears may be completely bitten off in human bite attacks. Cat bites are small and round with pointed cuspid tooth impressions due to the conical shape of these teeth. Claw scratches may also be noted in feline bites.[83] The forensic pathologist, of course, is well acquainted with the appearance of postmortem animal biting artefact as noted upon the deceased body.[84]

PROCEDURAL ASPECTS OF BITE MARK ANALYSIS
Examination of the Bite Mark on the Victim

Upon recognition of a bite mark injury, the forensic investigation should commence as soon as possible. Registration of the bite mark on a victim is one of the few areas in forensic pathology necessitating an immediate response at any hour of day or night, since just a few hours delay may mean the loss of potentially valuable points of indentation or areas of superficial skin contusion. With the passage of time, even postmortem, bite indentations may smooth out and minor contusions may fade. Ultraviolet or infrared illumination has been utilized to demonstrate faint areas of contusion not readily recognized using light of the visible wavelengths. Despite earlier comments regarding postmortem change, the passage of time in itself does not, by any means, negate the validity of the bite mark comparison. A well preserved body without the obvious effects of postmortem decomposition will possess minimal, if any, distortion of the bite mark in relation to the mark at the time of infliction. Many defense counselors will raise the issue of postmortem shrinkage of tissue as a means of discrediting the analysis; however, such changes in the preserved body are minimal and represent a lesser source of dimensional error than possible dimensional change related to distortion of the skin surface as a result of the pressures inherent to the act of biting.

Salivary Secretory Substance Retrieval

The first step in the bite mark examination is the swabbing of the involved skin surface to detect the possible presence of secretory antigens conveyed by the saliva of the biter. Approximately 80 percent of persons are *secretors;* and the basic, A, B and O blood group protein antigenic complexes, quite concentrated in saliva relative to blood, are present in the various body fluids of such persons. The detection of salivary secretory antigens may further implicate or eliminate a particular suspect in any given case. The actual test for secretory antigens is performed by the serology section of the crime laboratory. It is important that the responsible serologic laboratory workers be familiar with the methods employed so that erroneous data does not serve to complicate an otherwise acceptable bite mark comparison based upon the morphologic criteria. Different laboratories may also perform the serologic examination utilizing any one of several available methods. It is vital that the consultant dentist inquire beforehand to provide the test material in a manner consistent with the methodology of the laboratory concerned. The test for secretory substance should be implemented as soon as possible, for such antigens in saliva may break down rapidly due to the presence of proteolytic enzymes.

The bite mark saliva sample is acquired by swabbing the involved area in concentric fashion, utilizing a sterile cotton swab moistened with isotonic saline solution. The examiner should not handle the cotton end of the swab lest he contaminate it with his own sweat or skin secretion. The swab is then placed in a clean dry vial for transmission to the laboratory. The presence of dried saliva upon the bite does not necessarily obviate the detection of secretory substance.

In addition to a swab of the bitten surface, a control swab, used in similar fashion, should be applied to an unbitten skin surface of the victim. The intraoral saliva and a blood sample of the victim must also be procured for examination purposes.

The bite mark and control swabs should be used at the very outset of the examination prior to the removal of clothing and certainly prior to any wiping of the body surfaces for cleansing purposes. The examiner should keep in mind that any blood contamination of a so-called saliva sample will introduce error into the results. It is not inconceivable that prior orogenital sexual activity on the part of the deceased, contaminated by the ejaculate of the assailant, may confuse the secretory type of the victim. The victim's skin control swabs and blood type determination, however, should resolve any such discrepancy. Furthermore, the pathologist in such suspected cases should perform an oral smear to demonstrate spermatozoa.

If the bite mark swabs reveal an absence of detectable secretory substance, two possibilities exist:

1. The secretory substance is not detectable postmortem.
2. The biter is a nonsecretor.

It should be mentioned that the salivary secretory substance analysis in bite mark cases generally results in an absence of any detectable secretory antigen. This is to say that the percentage yield is low as a result of postmortem drying and the current methodology available for such determinations. Nevertheless, the test should be performed in every bite mark case.

If the bite mark swabs reveal a secretory type different than that of the deceased, the implication is that the biter was a secretor of the type discovered.

If the bite mark and control swabs disclose similar A, B and O secretory typing for both the victim and the area of bite mark, no conclusions can be drawn.

Registration of the Bite Mark

As stated earlier, the science of bite mark analysis involves a comparison of the bite mark with the dentition of the suspect. The registration of the bite mark is accomplished by one or both of the following methods: (1) the photographic method and (2) the impression method.

Both methods employ the use of models of the suspect's dentition for comparison with the recorded bite mark. The photographic method uses a photograph of the bite mark as a means of bite mark registration, while the impression method utilizes a rubber-base or silicone impression which is then converted to a model of the bite mark preferably made from plaster-of-paris. The characteristics of morphology and measurements of the recorded bite mark from either the photograph and/or the bite mark model are then compared with the corresponding features of the suspect's dentition. If possible and if known, the actual position of the body at the time of bite should be reconstructed when bite registration is effected. This statement is made to stress consideration of the possible alteration in arch morphology due to skin stretching.[85]

THE PHOTOGRAPHIC METHOD: Prior to the performance of the autopsy and following swabbing for saliva, the bite mark must be photographed *in situ,* and a rigid millimeter rule must be incorporated within the photograph positioned next to and adjacent to the plane of the bite mark. The ruler is an essential element because the eventual comparison of the mark with the suspect's dentition will be made using life-size models of his dentition. The incorporation of the ruler allows a life-size one-to-one enlargement or duplication of the bite mark negative to be made and thereby enables direct comparison by photograph or measurement with the life-size models of the suspect and with Aluwax® bites derived from the models. The film used should be suitable for both black and white as well as color photographs. Black and white photographs should be available for introduction as court evidence if an objection arises regarding inflammatory (to the jury) color photographs. In addition, black and white film allows finer resolution upon printing or enlargement. The color photographs can be used for the detailed comparison examination and show to advantage the gradation of pressure points and areas of contusion and abrasion as compared to a black and white photograph. Transparencies of the bite mark are also advisable for easy explanation to the court of the techniques employed. One should also take one photograph of the bite mark without a ruler to refute any claims that the ruler is covering other evidence.

It is best to use a camera producing 3¼-by-4-inch or 4-by-5-inch pictures rather than a 35mm camera since there is greater resolution in enlargements or duplications made with the larger negative. Oblique lighting may be employed to highlight any bite indentations.

If the bite mark has been inflicted upon a convex surface, such as the dome of the breast or the convexity of the arm, it may be helpful to take a separate photograph of each arch pattern since a single overhead photograph may distort the more distant anterior rim of each arch and the depth of field focus and subject curvature may alter the photographic reproduction. For optimal results, the film plane should be parallel to the plane of the bitten surface and the plane of the adjacent ruler.

An experienced photographer or a pathologist or dentist thoroughly knowledgeable with his camera equipment should perform the photographic techniques because a photographic failure may ruin or severely complicate the analysis.

THE IMPRESSION METHOD: While photographic registration of the bite mark should be done in every case, the impression method need only be applied if bite indentations are present within the skin surface. The value of the impression method rests upon the fact that bite mark indentations of the skin are exactly reproduced in the three-dimensional model; and thus, the dimension of depth is provided for comparison with the dentition of the suspect. It must be understood that at the time of bite mark injury, particular tooth mark indentations will always be present. The passage of time, however, results in a smoothing out of the tooth depressions. The latter phenomenon occurs as a result of edema due to injury, postmortem change and the inherent ability of the plastic skin, dermis and subdermal tissues to reconstitute the original contour of the body surface. At a later point in time only the tooth contusions (bruises) or less common tooth lacerations (tears in the skin) remain as hallmarks of the bite. Sebata[86] has stated that bite marks which do not break the skin surface will persist for as short an interval as three minutes or as long as twenty-four hours, depending upon the bite pressure applied. Harvey[87] has stated that face bites fade more quickly than bites upon other body areas and, further, that bite marks upon the male subject fade more rapidly than bites inflicted upon females.

Rubber base or silicone impression compounds should be applied to the bitten area and reinforced by stone after setting but prior to removal from the body surface. The stone backing preserves the general contour of the skin surface. A subsequent plaster positive of the rubber base impression can also be poured to create a facsimile of the mark indentations.

When both the photographic and impression methods are utilized in the analysis, the photographic workup should precede the application of impression-making materials to the skin surface. It is also advisable to take several rubber-base or silicone impressions, and if necessary, several plaster models of each impression can be made.

Preservation of the Bitten Tissue

Upon completion of the secretory substance swab examination, the photographic registration and the impression method (if indicated), it is ideal to remove the anatomic area of the bite mark for preservation as evidence and further examination if necessary. Before the decision is made to excise the bite mark from the body, it is best to be certain that the photographic registration is acceptable. This implies that rapid development, at least of the negatives, be carried out so that the analyst is assured of good quality photographs. Such a requisition may delay release of the body for some hours; however, it guarantees that vital evidence is not lost.

The above statement is made because once the tissue is removed from the body, depending upon the area of the bite, distortion of the bite mark is apt to occur. It is mandatory that the photographs and impressions be taken *in situ* and not after excision of the bite mark.

The pathologist should excise the bite mark exercising wide latitudes of tissue resection to minimize specimen distortion due to release of tissue tension and change in tissue elasticity. Such resection may require the removal of the entire underlying soft tissues to the bone or the removal of an entire breast. If the bite mark involves the cheek, forehead or neck area, the pathologist must exercise judgment regarding the value of retrieving the tissue specimen versus the wishes of next of kin for subsequent facial viewing at the funeral. Most laws covering the postmortem examination of deaths resulting from violence sanction the retention by the pathologist of any tissue specimen deemed necessary as medicolegal evidence. If the existing medical examiner law fails to include such a statement, the pathologist should contact the attorney general of the jurisdiction and clarify the issue prior to the removal of facial structures, an act which may be considered mutilation by the next of kin. If adequate photographs and impressions have been made, the pathologist may wish not to remove the bitten tissue; however, a question may later arise that can only be clarified by direct examination of the original specimen.

Upon removal of the bite mark tissue, the specimen should be retained and preserved in 10% formalin or Keiserling's solution. A tissue shrinkage of 10 to 20 percent is common with such preservatives, thereby obviating any future comparative measurements since the mark is no longer a life-size specimen.

Microscopic Examination of the Bite Mark

Following preservation and fixation of the bite mark, and upon satisfaction that the specimen itself can be incised, a histologic section of a contused segment of the bite mark should be examined microscopically to ascertain the time of the injury relative to the time of death. This should be done in every bite mark case to, in fact, establish with reasonable certainty that the bite occurred at the same time the fatal injury or injuries were inflicted.

Registration of the Dentition of the Victim

In instances where the anatomic position of the bite mark upon the victim is consistent with self-biting, dental impressions and models should be obtained of the victim's dentition. Such a precaution will forever dismiss the possibility, which may be raised in the future, that the deceased had bitten herself (himself). In cases where the suspected assailant is believed to have been bitten by the deceased, the registration of the victim's dentition may be necessary to relate the assailant to the crime.

Registration of Bite Marks from Objects Other than the Body

Numerous instances are on record of bite marks found in materials other than human tissue, especially within foodstuffs.[88-91] Due to the deterioration of certain foodstuffs as a result of environmental conditions, rapid processing of such bite mark evidence is of utmost importance. If a dentist is not readily available to examine the case, the investigating police personnel should not hesitate to contact a law enforcement tool mark examination laboratory since the techniques employed are similar to those utilized in certain tool mark comparison studies.

A plaster-of-paris or rubber base impression should be made of the bitten object, and a model of the original should then be constructed. The comparison between the morphology of the teeth of a criminal suspect and the bite features of the object is then made. A one-to-one photograph of the original foodstuff is advisable; however, generally speaking, the models (and photographs) of the bitten substance are sufficient for presentation of the points of comparison.

Hodson[92] has found that mixtures of alcohol and formalin are suitable for the preservation of apples. Once the original foodstuff has been processed it is also advisable to preserve the specimen by freezing or by placing in 10% formalin.

Registration of the Suspect's Dentition

Upon completion of the techniques of bite mark registration of the substance bitten, the attention of the analyst is then focused upon the biter. Several months may elapse before the suspect is located, in which case it is important to establish, in fact, that no alterations (extractions, etc.) of the suspect's dentition have occurred in the interim.

Of preliminary concern when confronted with the registration of the dentition of the suspect are the legal technicalities involved in obtaining the models of a suspect's teeth. In every instance, the analyst should have a court order issued by a governing judge or a legal consent form signed by the suspect giving permission to perform the necessary medicolegal examination. Either of the above must be in hand prior to the examination because

1. the dentist may be liable for assault upon the suspect if voluntary permission has not been granted in the absence of a court order and
2. evidence of this nature may not be admitted at the trial unless either of the above has been obtained prior to the retrieval of data.

Other legal aspects of bite mark evidence will be considered in a later section of this chapter.

The format of a legal consent form to be signed by the suspect is provided:

I, (name of suspect) , do hereby grant Dr. _____ , or persons under his direction, to examine, photograph and take impressions of my teeth. In addition, I hereby grant permission for this individual(s) to take saliva and blood samples. I fully understand that these measures are being instituted in connection with the investigation of the death of (name of deceased) .

Signed: _____ (suspect)

Witness: _____

Witness: _____

Date: _____

The first step in examination of the suspect is a charting of the dentition noting restorations, caries, extraction sites, incisal fractures, areas of rotation, etc. Photographs of the dentition should also be made including the anterior jaws in centric occlusion as well as the incisal aspects.

Several milliliters of saliva for secretory antigen analysis should be obtained and forwarded immediately to the serologic laboratory. Again, the particular laboratory must be consulted regarding the nature of the sample. Some facilities may prefer to work with a dried saliva sample on filter paper. Others may prefer a container of saliva after heat treatment to denaturize proteolytic enzymes which may destroy secretory antigens.

A blood sample of the suspect must also be obtained to establish his blood group. This is procured from an antecubital vein using proper blood-drawing technique.

The registration of the suspect's dentition is accomplished by obtaining models of the dentition of the suspect via alginate (Jeltrate®) impressions with subsequent stone models. One should keep in mind that reproduction of the incisal and occlusal surfaces is most important and the impression tray should not be so deeply seated that it distorts the cuspal or incisal surfaces of the canine teeth. The stone models should be poured immediately to eliminate any shrinkage in the alginate due to the passage of time.

With the suspect's models in hand, particular attention must be directed to the characteristics of the dental arches as well as specific features of individual teeth, especially those teeth considered to be involved in the bite mark pattern. The models should be verified as being representative of the dentition and free of disturbing discrepancies. Features such as the inter-jaw relationship, missing or carious teeth, the morphology of the incisal and/or occlusal aspects of the teeth and inter-tooth spacing should be noted. A centric wax bite should also be obtained for purposes of mounting the casts upon an articulator.

The next step in relating the dentition of the suspect of the bite mark involves the reproduction of the suspect's model bite characteristics upon a medium suitable for comparison with the photograph or model of the bite mark. The object is to derive a reproduction of the biting or pressure-inducing surfaces of the models and to compare the measurements and morphology of these surfaces with the corresponding bite mark areas of the skin or foodstuff. Several technical procedures have been effected by various investigators to achieve this comparison. Such procedures have been presented above under "General Considerations."

The author prefers to transfer the incisal/occlusal aspects of the articulated suspect's casts upon Aluwax®. Photographs printed at a one-to-one relation to the Aluwax® bite can then be used for direct comparison with the one-to-one photograph of the actual bite mark. Negatives of the wax bite photograph or color reversal film negatives of the wax bite can also be utilized for superimposition of the wax bite upon the actual mark photograph. A ruler, of course, must be included in every wax bite photograph to insure a one-to-one reproduction.

With the above data in hand, the analyst is prepared for the comparison phase of the bite mark analysis.

THE BITE MARK COMPARISON

It should again be mentioned and reemphasized that no single method for the analysis of bite mark evidence exists and that the particular method or methods employed depend upon the circumstances of the individual case and the preference of the analyst. The fact is that the methods of comparison speak for themselves as being a scientific study involving the comparison of a bite mark with a duplication of the expected bite contusion pattern of the suspect's dentition.

It should also be realized that bite marks may vary considerably from case to case in terms of the evidence at hand. A *good* bite mark is one that is characterized by variations of the following features:

1. a short time interval between the infliction of the bite injury and its registration,
2. the degree of force exerted and the resultant contusion-abrasion pattern and
3. the presence or absence of peculiarities of the dental arch.

Features inherent to an excellent bite mark would be a recent mark complete with tooth indentations capable of reproduction in an impression-making medium, definitive areas of contusion and the presence of specific peculiarities in the alignment or arrangement of the bite mark components. On the other hand, the absence of such ideal circumstances does not by any means eliminate the importance of the analysis. To be sure, bite marks having less than ideal criteria as stated above may still constitute more than enough data so that definitive conclusions regarding the comparison can be made.

In any bite mark comparison, the analyst must always remember that numerous variables exist in the imprint pattern of incisal and occlusal surfaces as effected upon human skin. To begin with, skin, unlike a wax bite, is an amazingly elastic medium capable of distortion due to pressure and anatomic position of the bitten part or in response to sucking action which may be inherent in the mechanics of bite injury. Varying degrees of skin tension (due to elastic fibers in the dermis) exist depending upon the relative position of the bitten area. This phenomenon of skin stretching or relaxation is vividly brought to mind if one reflects upon the distortion of self-applied stick-on tattoos, a fantasy commonly enjoyed by children. Devore[85] has formally reintroduced this concept as it applies to bite marks. Figure 61 discloses just such alterations in an imprint pattern. For this reason it is best, if possible, to reconstruct the actual body position at the time of bite injury. Figure 62 portrays an actual case where distortion resulted in an inconsistency in the comparison.

Another important concept that must be understood prior to the interpretation of a bite injury is that the bite mark injury is a result of biting

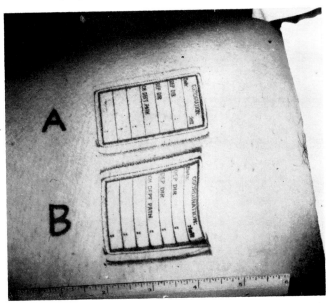

Figure 61. Application of a rectangular rubber stamp to the inner right thigh. At A, the stamp was applied without skin tension. Pressure upon the skin to the right of rectangle B at the time of application resulted in marked distortion.

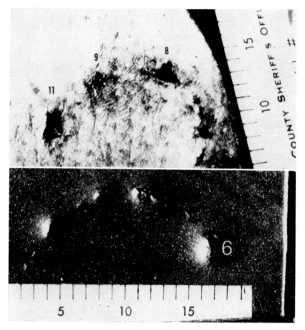

Figure 62. The inconsistency of the right side of the mark was attributed to skin stretching at the time of the bite. Note the deviation to the left of the area 6-7 of the mark (top) when compared to the wax bite (bottom).

force which spans a spectrum from minimal contact with the skin surface to a deep incised puncture wound which may penetrate to the underlying subcutaneous soft tissues. What is actually represented in the bite mark is the resultant residual injury to a body tissue due to the application of an unknown degree of biting pressure exerted at some point between bare contact to extreme clenching of the tissues. Each small area of injured skin will portray a gradation of tissue injury ranging from superficial abrasion to deep contusion or laceration depending upon the totality of forces acting on that area of tissue at the time of injury. Skin tissue is capable of varying degrees of deformation before an injury threshold is achieved; the injury is perceived as an abrasion (scrape of the epidermis), contusion (hemorrhage of the underlying dermis) or laceration (tear of the skin). The above explains why multiple test bites of the suspect's models into wax must be effected at differing degrees of pressure in an attempt to approximate an imprint pattern as noted in the bite mark registration. Invariably, considerably less pressure is required in wax (Aluwax®) to duplicate the injury pattern noted in the skin. The reason for this is that the skin absorbs considerable kinetic energy of bite forces prior to the inherent level of force necessary for resultant visible injury.

The concept of range of pressure required for injury also explains why, in many bite marks, only portions of an incisal surface of any particular tooth may be represented in the contusion pattern. Examination of the models of such suspect's arches will disclose that the tooth in question possesses a tapering or oblique incisal surface so that equal force is not delivered by the entire incisal surface.

While discussing the nature of the bite injury itself, it should be mentioned that the individual's susceptibility to injury may vary depending upon age, sex, site of the bite and the presence or absence of any natural disease which may increase any bleeding tendency. The elderly tend to bruise more easily than the young, and females more readily bruise than males. Common natural disease states which may lead to increased hemorrhaging with minimal injury include liver disease and various blood disorders.

The bite mark analyst must also bear in mind certain factors introduced into the comparison as a result of the mechanics of the bite when inflicted. Unlike the reproduction of the suspect's bite pattern as achieved in the laboratory, the actual biting of the victim is a dynamic (and not a static) process which involves complex movements of the jaws relative to each other as well as the possible movement of the victim in defense. Such activity of the dental arch-skin surface interface may result in areas of gliding abrasions and contusions which must be recognized as such.

In general terms, due to the diffusion of hemorrhage, a phenomenon which may persist postmortem, the area of contusion related to a particular tooth or portion thereof will be slightly larger than the surface area which caused the injury. This process of diffusion is responsible for the fading or haziness of the bite mark with time and the subsequent loss of what otherwise may represent an area of specificity.

The occurrence of sucking while biting may also introduce dimensional change in the interrelationship of the dental arch components due to obvious tenting of the bitten surface. The presence of a diffuse ovoid zone of subcutaneous hemorrhage within the central confines of the bite mark is suggestive of sucking activity.

Bite marks inflicted through clothing tend to reduce the degree of force on the tissues and may be responsible for the absence of particular tooth injuries. For example, maxillary lateral incisor injuries may be absent. In such a hypothetical example, one must not necessarily interpret the finding as indicative of absent lateral incisors.

The Conclusions of the Examiner

The dental expert is expected to answer the following questions regarding the comparison:

1. Can the suspect be excluded from consideration as having produced the bite mark?
2. If the suspect cannot be excluded, how specific are the points of comparison leading to the conclusion that the suspect alone could have produced the bite mark?

Of these two questions, the first is the easiest to answer and represents a vital contribution in itself because the comparison may confirm guilt or redirect the search for the suspect in question. The second question above, regarding the specificity of the comparison, encompasses the most difficult and controversial area within the realm of forensic odontology. The analyst is confronted with the problem of the individuality of the bite characteristics—the problem of specificity of the mark for the suspect alone to the exclusion of all other individuals.

The problem of specificity in the bite mark analysis results from the lack of a scientific core of basic data for comparison. The results of the bite mark comparison may indicate a perfect or reasonably perfect fit between the bite mark and a suspect's dentition; however, how can one be absolutely or even perhaps reasonably certain that no other individual could have produced a particular bite? Classified bite mark characteristics on large segments of the population are unavailable; therefore, an absolute scientific estimation of specificity regarding the particular bite mark/suspect comparison is not possible. The situation is comparable to the point in the distant past when the 100th set of fingerprints was classified. At that time, it was known that the set of prints did not match the ninety-nine others previously recorded, but it was not known if the set of prints were specific for only the one individual fingerprinted. Today, after categorizing 84 million sets of fingerprints in the United States, it can be stated with certainty that no two sets match. The present position of bite mark specificity is comparable to the 100th fingerprint case example. This is the problem that confronts the dental expert when he ponders the question of specificity. Due to the fact that the bite mark analyst cannot relate his findings to a classified body of knowledge regarding bite mark analyses, he finds difficulty in assessing a degree of probability or a realm of *reasonable dental certainty* concerning his formal opinion. It is only proper in the pursuit of truth regarding such important forensic evidence that this point be made clear to the prosecution, defense and jury. Obviously, however, any particular case may present unusual arch features which strongly indicate a particular mouth.

The above discussion of specificity must be seriously considered and never forgotten by the analyst. This especially applies to bite mark cases wherein subjective interpretation of the data exists. The author has personally handled a bite mark case in which it was established by the police investigation that one of two specific persons was responsible for the bite mark and death of the individual. Of many bite marks upon the body, only one was suitable for comparison studies (the others had faded to the point where tooth specificity was lost). The bite mark analyzed was of fair to good quality with a total of six lower and five upper anterior teeth represented. Despite the fact that only one of the suspects committed the bite, it was not possible to implicate either subject to the exclusion of the other. Both mouths were quite consistent with the bite mark. While it is true that an obvious discriminating feature between the subjects existed (marked rotation of an upper central incisor), this particular tooth failed to leave a distinct bite contusion. The perpetrator of the crime subsequently confessed to the bites, yet retrospectively, this examiner still could not implicate one mouth to the exclusion of the other. It is also interesting that the total circumstances surrounding the death incriminated the nonguilty subject rather than the confessor as having committed the crime. Had the eventual confessor not been considered a suspect, the dental evidence in this case would have implicated the nonguilty subject.

The forensic dentist attempts to enumerate the points of comparison between the bite mark and the models in an effort to enhance the specificity of the comparison procedure. The number of points of comparison will depend upon the circumstances of the bite mark. Such circumstances include the quality of the mark itself, the presence or absence of possible distortion induced by postmortem or positional change and the peculiarities of the mark as they pertain to the dentition of the suspect. It must be reiterated that human skin is a poor medium for registration of a bite mark. More points of comparison in the absence of inconsistencies or incompatibilities enable a more valid conclusion to be derived regarding any given suspect.

The author does not agree with those bite mark experts who only state that the *bite mark is consistent or not consistent* with a given suspect in the face of more incriminating specificity within the bite mark examination. He does not feel that such a blanket statement should categorically apply to all bite mark cases. While it is true that a poor quality bite mark possessing few measurable specific points of comparison may enable only such a *consistent* conclusion, many cases reveal further degrees of specificity with the connotation of being extremely consistent with the suspect's dentition depending upon the peculiarities noted. To withhold such additional information from the court lessens the degree of circumstantiality of the evidence and favors the suspect. The strength of the evidence must be indicated to the court. If one accepts the concept, on the basis of the earlier discussion, that one cannot precisely state the probability or degree of certainty inherent in his conclusions, it is, nevertheless, important to clarify the opinion by indicating the status of the findings regarding the weakness or strength of what must be regarded as evidence. The author feels that each case, depending upon the comparison results, should be indicated as weak, strong or extremely strong in discriminatory evidence against the suspect in question.

In summary, bite mark comparison results may represent varying degrees of incriminating evidence which must be so designated by the dental expert so that the court or jury can apply the weight of the evidence in proper perspective to the total circumstances surrounding the trial. The defense counsel may attempt to totally exclude the admission of bite mark evidence on the basis of its credibility. Such action merely eliminates a valuable segment of evidence offered to arrive at the truth. The methods of bite mark comparison are based on scientific principles as advanced as the current state of the art. Such evidence should not be suppressed if one wishes to pursue the totality that can be afforded by medicolegal evidence in the search of truth.

LEGAL ASPECTS OF BITE MARK CASES

Concomitant with the increased exposure of law enforcement agencies, the forensic pathologist and the legal profession to the science of bite mark analysis, an ever increasing number of bite mark cases are presently being recognized. Such awareness has also led to an increasing acceptance by the courts of both the admissibility of bite mark evidence as well as of the doctrine of court order which requires a suspect in a bite mark case to submit to dental examination for purposes of a bite mark comparison. Nevertheless, a potential legal problem may confront the investigating agency in its efforts to gain access to the dentition of a suspect. In his defense, the suspect may object to such an examination on the grounds that dental photographs, dental impressions and saliva samples represent techniques which may serve as evidence against him or as intrusions of privacy. Specifically, the suspect's counsel may invoke objection against the examination by claiming refuge under the protection of the Fourth or Fifth Amendments to the Constitution. Respectively, these amendments state that an individual has a right to be free of unreasonable searches and seizures and that a subject has a privilege not to incriminate himself.

Moncier and Hinnant[93] and, more recently, Dinkel[94] have researched the legal literature and have expressed opinions regarding interpretation of these amendments in relation to the bite mark suspect and consent for examination. The results of their research and their conclusions will be briefly presented.

Dinkel relates that he could not find a single recorded instance in which the constitutionality of compelling a suspect to submit to dental impressions has been litigated. By analogy, however, the general subject of body intrusion and search has been extensively litigated. To be sure, numerous courts have upheld the constitutionality of the submission of criminal suspects to comparison studies such as fingerprint analysis, photographs, police lineup identification, the acquisition of hair samples and voice prints as well as fingernail scrapings and handwriting exemplars.

Moncier and Hinnant expressly state that *dental printing* of a suspect would not be subject to the protection of the Fifth Amendment against self-incrimination. They cite the Supreme Court interpretation in *Schmerber v. California*[95] wherein blood was extracted from a subject for purposes of blood alcohol determination. The Court excluded this action as a violation of the Fifth Amendment because this privilege *protects an accused only from being compelled to testify against himself or otherwise provide the state with evidence of a testimonial or communicative nature*. In essence, an individual's right not to be a witness against himself applies to *communications*.[96] For example, lineup identification of suspects[97] and handwriting exemplars[98] have been ruled as not included in Fifth Amendment *communications*. The Supreme Court in *Schmerber v. California*[95] further noted that many identification procedures are not protected by the Fifth Amendment, stating that *both federal and state courts have usually held that it (the Fifth Amendment) offers no protection against compulsion to submit to fingerprinting, photographing or measurements*. Dinkel further cites the military case of *U.S. v. Culver*[99] wherein the Court of Military Review upheld the dentist's comparison of a tooth fragment with the accused's dentition by stating that such evidence (or communication) does not fall within the purview of the Fifth Amendment. Subsequent to the above-mentioned Schmerber decision, body intrusions limited to observations and comparison (such as identification procedures) are not testimonial or communicative in nature and are not applicable to the Fifth Amendment.

In the recent Connecticut case, *State v. Rice*[100] dental casts of a defendant in a bite mark case were obtained without prior consent. The defense motion to suppress such evidence was denied by the presiding judge who stated *police may take impressions of a suspect's teeth incidental to arrest when needed for evidence and such action does not violate the privilege against self-incrimination*.

In reference to the Fourth Amendment protection against unreasonable search and seizure, both Dinkel and Moncier and Hinnant again refer to the Schmerber decision.[95] The Court in Schmerber stated, "*The overriding function of the Fourth Amendment is to protect personal privacy and dignity against unwarranted intrusion by the State. . . . The Fourth Amendment's proper function is to constrain not against all intrusions as such but against intrusions which are not justified in the circumstances or which are made in an improper manner.*" Moncier and Hinnant cite the case of *U.S. v. Doe,*[101] wherein the Court ruled that *"handwriting and voice exemplars (represent areas wherein) no reasonable expectation of privacy exists."* They further add the case of *U.S.. v. Davis*[102] wherein the Court stated that fingerprints do not involve probing of an individual's private life and thoughts, nor can they be repeatedly used to harass the individual. Dinkel points out the case of *Katz v. U.S.*[103] wherein it was determined that one does not possess a reasonable expectation of privacy for his dentition as one's teeth are continually exposed to the public in addition to leaving bite impressions in foodstuffs bitten.

In summary, the conclusions forwarded by Moncier and Hinnant as well as Dinkel produce a series of legal decisions upon analogous circumstances which indicate that neither the Fourth nor the Fifth Amendments serve as substantial objections to the submission of a suspect to the dental examination for purposes of bite mark comparison. Specifically, Moncier and Hinnant concluded that a lawfully detained suspect could be subjected to dental examination without his consent or judicial authorization. A consenting individual may always be subjected to the examination. On the other hand, a forced examination upon a nonconsenting individual should be avoided prior to lawful arrest or judicial authorization.

BITE MARK CASE PRESENTATION

The following section illustrates the workup of a bite mark case. The victim was a 21-year-old female who died as a result of multiple stab wounds of the torso. A bite mark was noted on the lateral aspect of the left arm (Fig. 63). The bite mark circumscribed a centrally located knife wound with the bite contusions presenting much like a clockface. A color photograph of the injury is presented as the Frontispiece.

Figure 64 illustrates an enlargement of the bite mark. The slightly eccentric central incised wound is surrounded by a rather diffuse zone of subcutaneous bruising which is limited by the dental arch outlines. Such bruising suggests that sucking occurred while biting. Although the author believes that the stab wound served as a focus for the subsequent bite injury, such a statement cannot be made with any degree of certainty.

Initially, the examiner could not determine which dental arch related to which aspect of the bite mark. The absence of prominent anterior tooth contusions is unusual for bite mark cases; however, the open bite of the

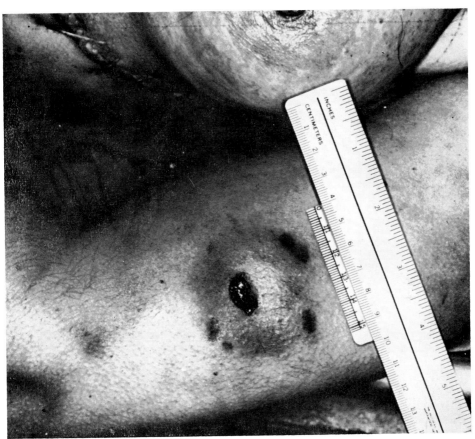

Figure 63. Original bite mark photograph utilized in the comparison procedure. The large ruler is superimposed upon the original photograph and indicates that the photograph is life-size or one-to-one. This is mandatory in any comparison with a suspect's dental models which, by definition, are life-size. AFIP Neg. No. 72-13451-5.

suspect and the possibility of sucking action as opposed to apprehension are explanations for this finding. To effect a preliminary screen of the mark and to establish the arch responsible for the respective portion of the mark, the following method was used:

1. The occlusal and incisal outlines of the suspect's upper and lower dental models were delineated. A one-to-one black and white photograph of each model was taken (Fig. 65).

2. Transparent acetate sheet film was then placed over the outlined model photographs, and acetate ink tracings of the arches were then drawn (Figs. 66 and 67).

3. The transparent tracings were then superimposed upon the original

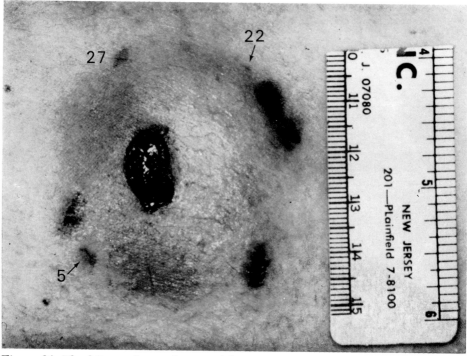

Figure 64. The bite mark reveals central bruising, suggestive of sucking action. The most specific characteristics of the mark include the diamond-shaped abrasion of 27, the prominent mesial incisal edge pressure contusion of 22 and the concave lingual cusp outline for tooth 5. AFIP Neg. No. 72-13451.

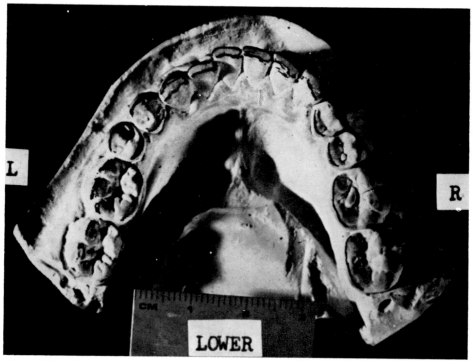

Figure 65. Life-size photograph of lower dental arch with pencil-outlined occlusal and incisal surfaces. The ruler is necessary to insure a one-to-one reproduction. AFIP Neg. No. 72-13451-2.

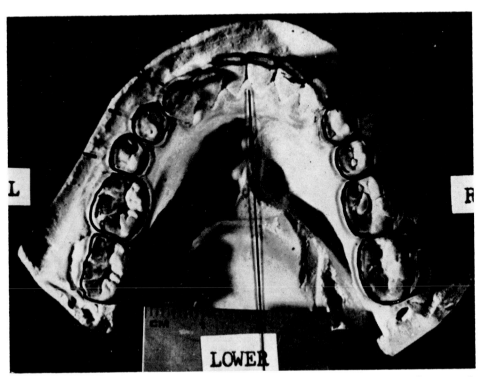

Figure 66. Acetate tracing drawn from photograph depicting outlines of expected pressure-inducing surfaces of all teeth. Note that the arch midline is also included. AFIP Neg. No. 72-13451-1.

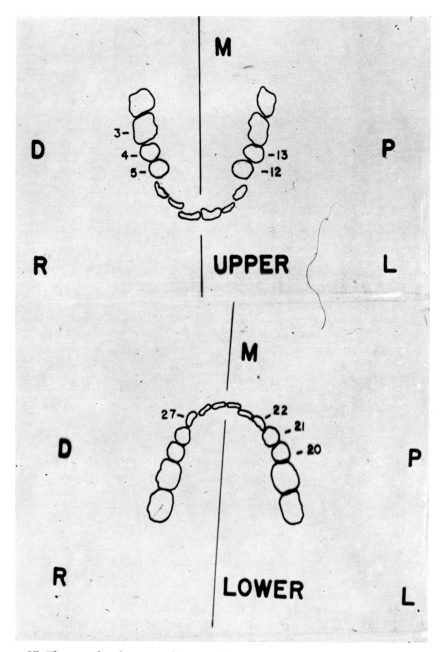

Figure 67. The completed acetate drawings for comparison by overlay upon the original bite mark photograph. The various letters indicate right and left, medial, distal and proximal; they provide rapid application of the tracings in the courtroom. AFIP Neg. No. 72-13451-9.

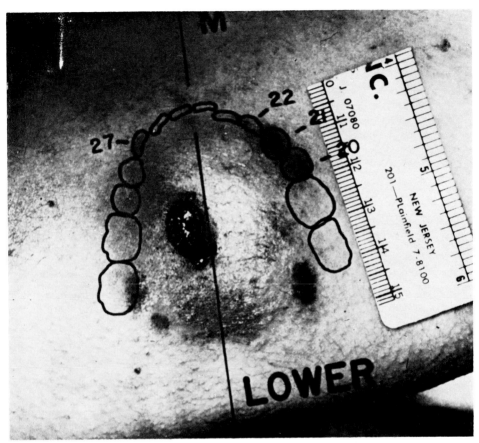

Figure 68. The lower tracing as applied to the medial arch of the mark. Note that the diamond-shaped defect of 27, the mesial incisal mark of 22 and the contusions for teeth 20 and 21 perfectly align. The points of specificity must be correlated with the dental models which provide a three-dimensional aspect of bite forces. AFIP Neg. 72-13451-12.

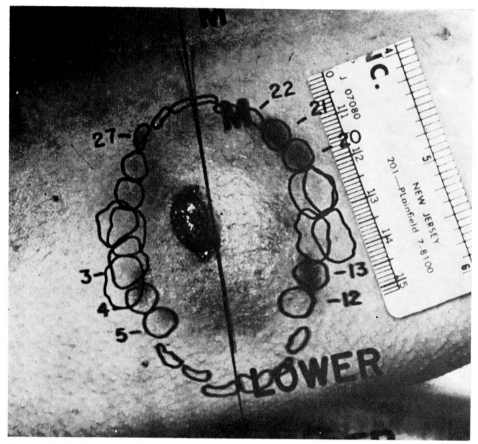

Figure 69. Both tracings have now been applied to the original photograph. Note that no contusions rest outside of the circles. The lingual cusp outline of 5 also corresponds perfectly with the tracing. The arch midlines also match. AFIP Neg. No. 72-13451-8.

one-to-one bite mark photograph, and the process of inclusion or exclusion of the suspect was initiated (Figs. 68 and 69).

The above procedure established that the subject could certainly not be excluded from producing the bite mark in question. The tracings also indicated that the medial bite mark was a result of the mandibular arch and that the lateral mark was due to the maxillary dentition. This finding corroborated the investigation at the scene of death where it appeared that the assailant leaned across the body of the deceased from right to left and inflicted the arm bite. Furthermore, the autopsy examination also disclosed that the knife wounds were inflicted from the right of the deceased.

To further elaborate the specific incisal and occlusal pressure imprints of the suspects' dental models, the models were mounted in an articulator, and wax bites in Aluwax® were taken (Fig. 70). In this way particular points for measurement between specific contusions could be established. The measurements between specific points in the wax as compared to the original photograph were practically identical. (In subsequent bite mark cases, the author has utilized negatives of wax bite photographs and superimposed these upon the original bite mark photographs. This method enables direct comparison of the bite contusions.)

Subsequent histologic sections of the bite injury indicated that the bite mark occurred at about the time of death.

The summary of the above bite mark analysis concluded as follows:

1. Fifteen points of exact comparison existed between the dental models and the bite mark. There were no incompatibilities.

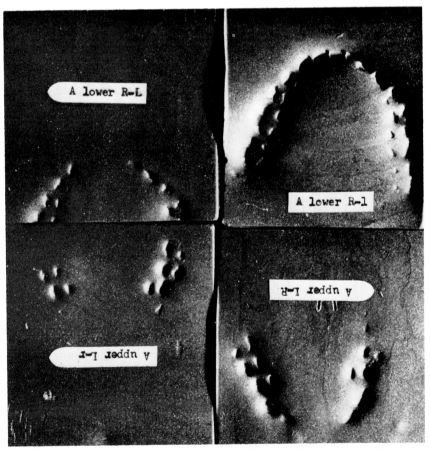

Figure 70. A pair of wax bites taken at differing degrees of pressure are shown side by side. Notice the absence of anterior tooth prints due to the peculiar open bite as noted on the articulator (not shown). It is important to take multiple wax bites at varying pressures in an attempt to approximate the degree of injury imparted to the tissues. AFIP Neg. No. 72-13451.

2. The assailant's lower jaw was in contact with the inner aspect of the arm; the upper jaw contacted the outer surface of the arm.

3. The bite mark occurred at about the time of death.

The opinion regarding the analysis was expressed as follows: *The bite mark analysis indicated that there was absolutely no doubt that the individual from whom the models were made would be expected to produce a bite mark pattern identical to the one noted on the arm of the victim.* Upon subsequent court testimony the opinion was expanded by stating that the mark was extremely consistent with the mouth of the suspect to the exclusion of others; however, it could not be stated with absolute certainty whether anyone else could have inflicted the bite injury.

BIBLIOGRAPHY

1. Davis, J. M., Sevien, F. A. C., and Feegel, J. R.: Investigative powers of the medical examiner in the light of Rupp versus Jackson. *J Forensic Sci*, 17:181, 1972.
2. Luke, J., Sturner, W., and Petty, C.: The status of forensic pathology in the United States today. *Forensic Sci Gazette (South W Inst Forensic Sci)*, 1:3, July 1970.
3. Kornblum, R. N., and Fisher, R. S.: *A Compendium of State Medico-Legal Investigative Systems.* Baltimore, Maryland Medical-Legal Foundation, May 1972.
4. Haines, D. H.: Dental identification in the Stockport air disaster. *Br Dent J 123:* 336, 1967.
5. Rosenbluth, E. S.: A legal identification. *Dental Cosmos*, 44:1029, 1902.
6. Grant, E. A., Prendergast, W. K., and White, E. A.: Dental identification in the Noronic disaster. *J Can Dent Assoc*, 18:3, 1952.
7. Knott, N. J.: Identification by the teeth of casualties in the Aberfan disaster. *Br Dent J, 122:*144, 1967.
8. Kerley, E. R.: Age determination of bone fragments. *J Forensic Sci, 14:*59, 1969.
9. Sopher, I. M.: The role of the forensic pathologist in arson and related investigations. *FBI Law Enforcement Bull, 41:*8, September 1972.
10. Teare, D.: Postmortem examinations on air crash victims. *Br Med J, 4733:*707, 1951.
11. Armed Forces Institute of Pathology (files of Aerospace Pathology Branch): Honolulu, Hawaii, Brittania CF-C2B aircraft accident, 1962. (Unpublished data.)
12. Keiser-Nielsen, S.: Dental investigation in mass disasters. *J Dent Res, 42:*303, 1963.
13. Salley, J. J., Filipowicz, F. J., and Karnitschnig, H. N.: Dental identification of mass disaster victims. *J Am Dent Assoc, 66:*827, 1963.
14. Fisher, R. S.: Elkton, Maryland Boeing 707 aircraft accident, 1963. (Unpublished data.)
15. Blair, E.: Identification of the casualties in the Kaimai air disaster. *NZ Dent J, 60:*151, 1964.
16. Stevens, P. J., and Tarlton, S. W.: Medical investigation in fatal aircraft accidents —the role of dental evidence. *Br Dent J, 120:*263, 1966.
17. Harmeling, B. L., Schuh, E., and Humphreys, H. S.: Dental identification of bodies in a major disaster. *Arkansas Dent J, 37:*12, 1966.
18. Haines, D. H.: Dental identification in the Stockport air disaster. *Br Dent J, 123:* 336, 1967.
19. Armed Forces Institute of Pathology (files of Aerospace Pathology Branch): Boone County, Kentucky Convair 880 aircraft accident, 1967. (Unpublished data.)
20. Van Wyk, C. W., Kemp, V. D., and Bukofzer, H.: The role of dental identification in the Windhoek aircrash. *Medicolegal J, 37:*79, 1969.

21. Petersen, K. B., and Kogon, S. L.: Dental identification in the Woodbridge disaster. *J Can Dent Assoc, 7*:275, 1971.
22. Luntz, L. L., and Luntz, P.: Dental identification of disaster victims by a dental disaster squad. *J Forensic Sci, 16*:63, 1972.
23. Haines, D. H.: Dental identification in the Rijeka air disaster. *Forensic Sci, 1*:313, 1972.
24. Stevens, P. J., and Tarlton, S. W.: Identification of mass casualties: Experience in four civil air disasters. *Med Sci Law, 3*:154, 1963.
25. Knott, N. J.: Identification by the teeth of casualties in the Aberfan disaster. *Br Dent J, 122*:144, 1967.
26. Ashley, K. F.: Identification of children in a mass disaster by estimation of dental age. *Br Dent J, 129*:167, 1970.
27. Mason, J. K.: Oral presentation at the Aerospace Pathology Course, Armed Forces Institute of Pathology, Washington, D.C., 1972.
28. Armed Forces Institute of Pathology (files of Aerospace Pathology Branch): Boston, Massachusetts, Electra aircraft accident, 1960. (Unpublished data.)
29. Armed Forces Institute of Pathology (files of Aerospace Pathology Branch): Lake Tahoe, Nevada, Constellation aircraft accident, 1964. (Unpublished data.)
30. Armed Forces Institute of Pathology (files of Aerospace Pathology Branch): Portland, Oregon, DC-9 aircraft accident, 1966. (Unpublished data.)
31. Armed Forces Institute of Pathology (files of Aerospace Pathology Branch): Urbana, Ohio, midair aircraft accident, 1967. (Unpublished data.)
32. Armed Forces Institute of Pathology (files of Aerospace Pathology Branch): Blossburg, Pennsylvania, BAC-111 aircraft accident, 1967. (Unpublished data.)
33. Sopher, I. M., and Angel, J. L.: Twenty-seven years later—the identification of seventeen air crash victims. (In preparation.)
34. Luntz, L. L.: A dentist puts teeth into the law. *Hartford Courant*, December 26, 1965.
35. Grant, E. A., Prendergast, W. K., and White, E.A.: Dental identification in the Noronic disaster. *J Can Dent Assoc, 18*:3, 1952.
36. Sopher, I. M., and Spitz, W. U.: Problems encountered in the dental identification of a mutilated body. *J Am Dent Assoc 83*:168, 1971.
37. Tattersall, W. R.: Identification by teeth and jaws—a survey. *Dental Record, 67*:66, 1947.
38. Identified by tooth. John Wilkes Booth's body recognized three years after death. *Am Dent J, 2*:477, 1903.
39. Scott, D. B.: Dental evidence in identification and criminology. In Gradwohl, R. B. H. (Ed.): *Legal Medicine*. St. Louis, Mosby, 1954, p. 470.
40. Gustafson, G.: *Forensic Odontology*. London, Staples Press, 1966, pp. 183-187.
41. Taber, L. B.: Denture-wearing celebrities. *J Calif State Dent Assoc, 29*:201, 1953.
42. Identification by the teeth. *Dental Advertiser, 22*:15, 1891.
43. Amoëdo, O.: The role of the dentists in the identification of the victims of the catastrophe of the Bazar de la Charité, Paris, May 4, 1897. *Dental Cosmos, 39*:905, 1897.
44. The Iroquois Fire. *Am Dent J, 3*:139, 1904.
45. Cleland, J. B.: Teeth and bites in history, literature, forensic medicine and otherwise. *Aust Dent J, 48*:107, 1944.
46. Bezymenski, L.: *The Death of Adolph Hitler*. New York, HarBrace J, 1968.
47. Sognnaes, R. F.: Dental identification of Hitler's deputy Martin Bormann. *J Am Dent Assoc, 86*:305, 1973.

48. Sognnaes, R. F., and Ström, F.: The odontological identification of Adolph Hitler. *Acta Odontol Scand, 31:*43, 1973.

49. Ström, F.: Dental aspects of forensic medicine. *Int Dent J, 4:*527, 1954.

50. Shafer, W. G., Hine, M. K., and Levy, B. M.: *Oral Pathology.* Philadelphia, Saunders, 1958, pp. 462-467.

51. Harvey, W.: Identity by teeth and the marking of dentures. *Br Dent J, 121:*334, 1966.

52. Jerman, A. C.: Denture identification. *J Am Dent Assoc, 80:*1358, 1970.

53. Shafer, W. G., Hine, M. K., and Levy, B. M.: *Oral Pathology.* Philadelphia, Saunders, 1958, pp. 114-116.

54. Keiser-Nielsen, S.: Geographic factors in forensic odontology. *Int Dent J, 15:*343, 1965.

55. Bang, G.: Factors of importance in dental identification: Five case reports. *Forensic Sci, 1:*91, 1972.

56. Lasker, C. W., and Lee, M. C.: Racial traits in human teeth. *J Forensic Sci, 2:*401, 1957.

57. Aitchison, J.: Some racial differences in human skulls and jaws. *Br Dent J, 116:* 25, 1964.

58. Hunt, E. E., Jr., and Gleiser, I.: The estimation of age and sex of preadolescent children from bones and teeth. *Am J Phys Anthropol, 13:*479, 1955.

59. Krogman, W. M.: *The Human Skeleton in Forensic Medicine.* Springfield, Thomas, 1962.

60. Stewart, T. D.: New developments in evaluating evidence from the skeleton. *J Dent Res, 42:*264, 1963.

61. Hurme, V. O.: Time and sequence of tooth eruption. *J Forensic Sci, 2:*377, 1957.

62. Hurme, V. O.: Standards of variations in the eruption of the first six permanent teeth. *Child Dev, 19:*213, 1948.

63. Falkner, F.: Deciduous tooth eruption. *Arch Dis Child, 32:*386, 1957.

64. Kraus, B. S.: Calcification of the human decidous teeth. *J Am Dent Assoc, 59:* 1128, 1959.

65. Stack, M. V.: Forensic estimation of age in infancy by gravimetric observations of the developing dentition. *J Forensic Sci Soc, 1:*49, 1960.

66. Boyde, A.: Estimation of age at death of young human skeletal remains from incremental lines in the dental enamel. *Proc 3rd International Meeting in Forensic Immunology, Medicine, Pathology and Toxicology.* London, April 16-24, 1963.

67. Miles, A. E. W.: The assessment of age from the dentition. *Proc R Soc Med, 51:* 1057, 1958.

68. Gustafson, G.: *Forensic Odontology.* London, Staples Press, 1966, p. 111.

69. Massler, M., and Schour, I.: The development of the human dentition. *J Am Dent Assoc, 28:*1153, 1941.

70. Miles, A. E. W.: Dentition in the estimation of age. *J Dent Res, 42:*255, 1963.

71. Brauer, J. C., and Badahur, M. A.: Variations in calcification and eruption of the deciduous and permanent teeth. *J Am Dent Assoc, 24:*1373, 1942.

72. Garn, S. M., Lewis, A. D., and Polacheck, D. L.: Variability of tooth formation. *J Dent Res, 38:*135, 1959.

73. Moorrees, C. F. S., Fanning, E. A., and Hunt, E. E., Jr.: Age variation of formation stages for ten permanent teeth. *J Dent Res, 42:*1490, 1963.

74. Fanning, E. A.: A longitudinal study of tooth formation and root resorption. *NZ Dent J, 57:*202, 1961.

75. Nolla, C. M.: The development of the permanent teeth. *J Dent Child, 27:*254, 1960.

76. Gustafson, G.: *Forensic Odontology.* London, Staples Press, 1966, pp. 118-140.

77. Nalbandian, J., and Sognnaes, R. F.: Structural age changes in human teeth. In Shock, N. W. (Ed.): *Aging Symposia: American Association for Advancement of Science.* Baltimore, Horn-Shafer, 1960, pp. 367-382.

78. Ström, F.: Investigations of bite marks. *J Dent Res, 42:*312, 1963.

79. Buhtz and Erhardt: In Gustafson, G.: *Forensic Odontology.* London, Staples Press, 1966, p. 156.

80. Morgen, H.: In Gustafson, G.: *Forensic Odontology.* London, Staples Press, 1966, p. 156.

81. Furness, J.: A new method for the identification of teeth marks in cases of assault and homicide. *Br Dent J, 124:*261, 1968.

82. Levine, L.: Forensic odontology today—a new forensic science. *FBI Law Enforcement Bull, 41:*6, August 1972.

83. Gustafson, G.: *Forensic Odontology.* London, Staples Press, 1966, pp. 143-144.

84. Spitz, W. U., and Fisher, R. S.: *Medicolegal Investigation of Death.* Springfield, Thomas, 1973, pp. 29-30.

85. DeVore, D. T.: Bite marks for identification?—a preliminary report. *Med Sci Law, 11:*144, 1971.

86. Sebata, M.: Medicolegal studies on bite marks. *Bull Tokyo Dent Coll, 4:*83, 1963.

87. Harvey, W., Butler, O., Furness, J., and Laird, R.: The Biggar murder. *J Forensic Sci Soc, 8:*188, 1968.

88. Furuhata, T., and Yamamoto, K.: *Forensic Odontology.* Springfield, Thomas, 1967, pp. 99-102.

89. Cleland, J. B.: Teeth and bites in history, literature, forensic medicine and otherwise. *Aust Dent J, 48:*107, 1944.

90. Cowley, J. O.: Don't bite more than you can chew. *Br Dent J, 96:*84, 1954.

91. Layton, J. J.: Identification from a bite mark in cheese. *J Forensic Sci Soc, 6:*76, 1966.

92. Hodson, J.: Forensic odontology and its role in the problems of the police and the forensic pathologist. *Med Sci Law, 10:*247, 1970.

93. Moncier, H. S., and Hinnant, M. B.: A study on bite marks. Washington, D.C., George Washington University Department of Forensic Sciences, 1972. Graduate thesis.

94. Dinkel, E. H.: The use of bite mark evidence as an investigative aid. *J Forensic Sci, 19:*535, 1974.

95. *Schmerber v. California,* 384 U.S. 757 (1966).

96. *Miranda v. Arizona,* 384 U.S. 436, 16 L.Ed. 2d 694, 6 S.Ct. 1602 (1966).

97. *Stoval v. Kemp,* 355 F. 2d 731 (2d Cir. 1966), cert. denied 384 U.S. 1000, 16 L.Ed. 2d 1014.

98. *Griffin v. California,* 388 U.S. 263 (1967).

99. *U.S. v. Culver,* 44 C.M.R. 564 (ACM 1971).

100. *State v. Rice,* 41 L.W. 4180 (1973).

101. *U.S. v. Doe* (Appeal of Schwartz), 2nd Circuit Court of Appeals, March 28, 1972, 11 Cr.L. 2047.

102. *U.S. v. Davis,* 394 U.S. 721, 89 S.Ct. 1394.

103. *Katz v. U.S.,* 389 U.S. 347.

INDEX

157